Praise for The Mindful Self-Compassion Workbook

"Drs. Neff and Germer have led the field in researching and articulating the transformative practices of Mindful Self-Compassion, and tens of thousands of people have been trained in their approach. Now you have in your hands a workbook that can guide your journey into profound healing and freedom; it provides a pathway that is accessible, clear, and rich in its depth. Please give yourself the gift of this book and share it with others—these teachings will serve many awakening hearts."
—*Tara Brach, PhD, author of* Radical Acceptance *and* True Refuge

"From their extensive insight and experience, Drs. Neff and Germer provide a friendly, easy-to-use workbook. Its powerful exercises will help you uncover your innate capacity to hold yourself—and the world around you—with compassion. Whether or not you take a formal Mindful Self-Compassion course, using this workbook can effect profound change in your life."
—*Sharon Salzberg, author of* Lovingkindness *and* Real Love

"Mindful Self-Compassion has made me far more resilient—when a storm hits, I float on the surface of the rough sea and wait for it to pass, rather than thrashing around trying to outswim it. I am able to find a nugget of joy every day, no matter how small. This workbook encourages a deeper understanding and experience of MSC. I recommend it to everyone."
—*Heather R., Hampshire, United Kingdom*

"Drs. Neff and Germer are the world's leading authorities on self-compassion. They show readers in simple, down-to-earth steps how to become more confident, less self-critical, and kinder to themselves. It feels like they are with you as warm and wise guides in every page of this book. Truly a gem."
—*Rick Hanson, PhD, author of* Resilient

THE MINDFUL SELF-COMPASSION WORKBOOK

Also from Kristin Neff and Christopher Germer

FOR GENERAL READERS

The Mindful Path to Self-Compassion:
Freeing Yourself from Destructive Thoughts and Emotions
Christopher Germer

FOR PROFESSIONALS

Mindfulness and Psychotherapy, Second Edition
*Edited by Christopher Germer, Ronald D. Siegel,
and Paul R. Fulton*

Teaching the Mindful Self-Compassion Program: A Guide for Professionals
(forthcoming)
Christopher Germer and Kristin Neff

Wisdom and Compassion in Psychotherapy:
Deepening Mindfulness in Clinical Practice
Christopher Germer and Ronald D. Siegel

The Mindful Self-Compassion Workbook

A PROVEN WAY TO ACCEPT YOURSELF, BUILD INNER STRENGTH, AND THRIVE

Kristin Neff, PhD
Christopher Germer, PhD

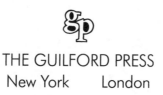

THE GUILFORD PRESS
New York   London

Published by The Guilford Press
A Division of Guilford Publications, Inc.
370 Seventh Avenue, Suite 1200, New York, NY 10001
www.guilford.com

Library of Congress Cataloging-in-Publication Data

Names: Neff, Kristin, author. | Germer, Christopher K., author.
Title: The mindful self-compassion workbook : a proven way to accept yourself, build inner strength, and thrive / Kristin Neff and Christopher Germer.
Description: New York, NY : Guilford Press, [2018] | Includes bibliographical references and index.
Identifiers: LCCN 2018011237 | ISBN 9781462535651 (hardcover : alk. paper) | ISBN 9781462526789 (pbk. : alk. paper)
Subjects: LCSH: Self-acceptance. | Compassion. | Security (Psychology)
Classification: LCC BF575.S37 N443 2018 | DDC 158.1/3—dc23
LC record available at https://lccn.loc.gov/2018011237

Acknowledgments

Although the authors of this book started developing Mindful Self-Compassion (MSC) in 2010, it is now a project of the worldwide community of MSC practitioners, teachers, and researchers, and we find ourselves in the enviable position of gathering their cumulative wisdom and integrating it into the training program you have in your hands. Our hope is that MSC will continually evolve as we learn together the subtle art of bringing compassion into the world, starting with kindness toward ourselves. To this end, we give thanks to the innumerable people whose voices are contained in the pages of this book.

We have also had the good fortune to live at a time when compassion practice and science are no longer separate subjects and where the wisdom of East and West is merging. This convergence is unprecedented in human history. We are therefore deeply grateful for luminaries who had the courage and vision to build these bridges, such as the Dalai Lama, Jon Kabat-Zinn, Sharon Salzberg, Jack Kornfield, Richie Davidson, Sara Lazar, Tania Singer, Pema Chödrön, Thupten Jinpa, Tara Brach, Daniel Siegel, Rick Hanson, and Paul Gilbert, to name just a few. Their efforts have paved the way for our own—bringing self-compassion training into mainstream society.

Right from the start, we had close colleagues who saw the value in self-compassion and joined our efforts in a variety of selfless ways. They included Michelle Becker, Steve Hickman, Christine Brähler, Susan Pollak, Pittman McGehee, Kristy Arbon, Lienhard Valentin, Wibo Koole, Hilde Steinhauser, Judith Soulsby, Vanessa Hope, Hailan Guo, Seogwang Snim, Marta Alonso Maynar, Dawn MacDonald, and Micheline St. Hilaire. Steve and Michelle, in particular, launched our MSC teacher training initiative in 2014 through the University of California, San Diego, and have collaboratively helped us develop the unique pedagogy that you will find in this book—self-compassion training that is safe and effective for a wide range of different people. It is our hope that readers who notice changes in their own lives through using this workbook will consider attending an actual MSC program and have a chance to interact with our talented, trained teachers who are the lifeblood of MSC. (You can find a local course at *www.centerformsc.org.*)

This book would not exist if not for the ardent support of Kitty Moore, our dear Senior Editor at The Guilford Press, who has been trying to make the world a better place for the past few decades. We are also grateful to Christine Benton, developmental editor, who read every word of this workbook for content and style to make it as readable and user-friendly as possible.

Finally, over the coming years we hope to pay back the generosity and understanding of our nearest and dearest, in particular Kristin's son, Rowan, and Chris's life partner, Claire. May their kind hearts be found by the reader in the pages of this book.

Contents

Purchasers of this book can download audio files to complement
some of the exercises at *www.guilford.com/neff-materials*
for personal use (see page 206 for details).

HOW TO USE THIS WORKBOOK

Most of the MSC curriculum is contained in this workbook, in an easy-to-use format that will help you start to be more self-compassionate right away. Some people who use this workbook will be currently taking an MSC course, some may want to refresh what they previously learned, but for many people this will be their first experience with MSC. This workbook is designed to also be a stand-alone pathway for you to learn the skills you need to be more self-compassionate in daily life. It follows the general structure of the MSC course, with the chapters organized in a carefully sequenced manner so the skills build upon one another. Each chapter provides basic information about a topic followed by practices and exercises that allow you to experience the concepts firsthand. Most of the chapters also contain illustrations of the personal experiences of participants in the MSC course, to help you know how the practices may play out in your life. These are composite illustrations that don't compromise the privacy of any particular participant, and the names are not real. In this book, we also alternate between masculine and feminine pronouns when referring to a single individual. We have made this choice to promote ease of reading as our language continues to evolve and not out of disrespect toward readers who identify with other personal pronouns. We sincerely hope that all will feel included.

We recommend that you go through the chapters in order, giving the time needed in between to do the practices a few times. A rough guideline would be to practice about 30 minutes a day and to do about one or two chapters per week. Go at your own pace, however. If you feel you need to go more slowly or spend extra time on a particular topic, please do so. Make the program your own. If you are interested in taking the MSC course in person from a trained MSC teacher, you can find a program near you at *www.centerformsc.org*. Online training is also available. For professionals who want to learn more about the theory, research, and practice of MSC, including how to teach self-compassion to clients, we recommend reading the MSC professional training manual, to be published by The Guilford Press in 2019.

The ideas and practices in this workbook are largely based on scientific research (notes at the back of the book point to the relevant research). However, they are also based on our experience teaching thousands of people how to be more self-compassionate. The MSC program is itself an organic entity, continuing to evolve as we and our participants learn and grow together.

Also, while MSC isn't therapy, it's very therapeutic—it will help you access the resource of self-compassion to meet and transform difficulties that inevitably emerge as we live our lives. However, the practice of self-compassion can sometimes activate old wounds, so if you have a history of trauma or are currently having mental health challenges, we recommend that you complete this workbook under the supervision of a therapist.

Tips for Practice

As you go through this workbook, it's important to keep some points in mind to get the most out of it.

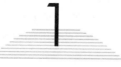

What Is Self-Compassion?

Self-compassion involves treating yourself the way you would treat a friend who is having a hard time—even if your friend blew it or is feeling inadequate, or is just facing a tough life challenge. Western culture places great emphasis on being kind to our friends, family, and neighbors who are struggling. Not so when it comes to ourselves. Self-compassion is a practice in which we learn to be a good friend to ourselves when we need it most—to become an inner ally rather than an inner enemy. But typically we don't treat ourselves as well as we treat our friends.

> *Through self-compassion we become an inner ally instead of an inner enemy.*

The golden rule says "Do unto others as you would have them do unto you." However, you probably don't want to do unto others as you do unto yourself! Imagine that your best friend calls you after she just got dumped by her partner, and this is how the conversation goes.

"Hey," you say, picking up the phone. "How are you?"

"Terrible," she says, choking back tears. "You know that guy Michael I've been dating? Well, he's the first man I've been really excited about since my divorce. Last night he told me that I was putting too much pressure on him and that he just wants to be friends. I'm devastated."

You sigh and say, "Well, to be perfectly honest, it's probably because you're old, ugly, and boring, not to mention needy and dependent. And you're at least 20 pounds overweight. I'd just give up now, because there's really no hope of finding anyone who will ever love you. I mean, frankly you don't deserve it!"

Would you ever talk this way to someone you cared about? Of course not. But strangely, this is precisely the type of thing we say to ourselves in such situations—or worse. With self-compassion, we learn to speak to ourselves like a good friend. "I'm so sorry. Are you okay? You must be so upset. Remember I'm here for you and I deeply appreciate you. Is there anything I can do to help?"

Although a simple way to think about self-compassion is treating yourself as you would treat a good friend, the more complete definition involves three core elements that we bring to bear when we are in pain: self-kindness, common humanity, and mindfulness.

Self-Kindness. When we make a mistake or fail in some way, we are more likely to beat ourselves up than put a supportive arm around our own shoulder. Think of all the generous, caring people you know who constantly tear themselves down (this may even be you). Self-kindness counters this tendency so that we are as caring toward ourselves as we are toward others. Rather than being harshly critical when noticing personal shortcomings, we are supportive and encouraging and aim to protect ourselves from harm. Instead of attacking and berating ourselves for being inadequate, we offer ourselves warmth and unconditional acceptance. Similarly, when external life circumstances are challenging and feel too difficult to bear, we actively soothe and comfort ourselves.

> *Theresa was excited. "I did it! I can't believe I did it! I was at an office party last week and blurted out something inappropriate to a coworker. Instead of doing my usual thing of calling myself terrible names, I tried to be kind and understanding. I told myself, 'Oh well, it's not the end of the world. I meant well even if it didn't come out in the best way.'"*

Common Humanity. A sense of interconnectedness is central to self-compassion. It's recognizing that all humans are flawed works-in-progress, that everyone fails, makes mistakes, and experiences hardship in life. Self-compassion honors the unavoidable fact that life entails suffering, for everyone, without exception. While this may seem obvious, it's so easy to forget. We fall into the trap of believing that

The Three Elements of Self-Compassion

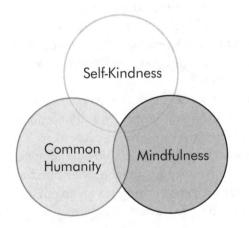

things are "supposed" to go well and that something has gone wrong when they don't. Of course, it's highly likely—in fact inevitable—that we'll make mistakes and experience hardships on a regular basis. This is completely normal and natural.

But we don't tend to be rational about these matters. Instead, not only do we suffer, we feel isolated and alone in our suffering. When we remember that pain is part of the shared human experience, however, every moment of suffering is transformed into a moment of connection with others. The pain I feel in difficult times is the same pain you feel in difficult times. The circumstances are different, the degree of pain is different, but the basic experience of human suffering is the same.

Theresa continued: "I remembered that everyone has a slip of the tongue sometimes. I can't expect to say the right thing at every moment. It's only natural that these things happen."

Mindfulness. Mindfulness involves being aware of moment-to-moment experience in a clear and balanced manner. It means being open to the reality of the present moment, allowing all thoughts, emotions, and sensations to enter awareness without resistance or avoidance (we will be delving more deeply into mindfulness in Chapter 6).

Why is mindfulness an essential component of self-compassion? Because we need to be able to turn toward and acknowledge when we're suffering, to "be" with our pain long enough to respond with care and kindness. While it might seem that suffering is blindingly obvious, many people don't acknowledge how much pain they're in, especially when that pain stems from their own self-criticism. Or when confronted with life challenges, people often get so caught up in problem-solving mode that they don't pause to consider how hard it is in the moment. Mindfulness counters the tendency to avoid painful thoughts and emotions, allowing us to face the truth of our experience, even when it's unpleasant. At the same time, mindfulness prevents us from becoming absorbed by and "overidentified" with negative thoughts or feelings, from getting caught up and swept away by our aversive reactions. Rumination narrows our focus and exaggerates our experience. Not only did I fail, *"I am a failure."* Not only was I disappointed, *"my life is disappointing."* When we mindfully observe our pain, however, we can acknowledge our suffering without exaggerating it, allowing us to take a wiser and more objective perspective on ourselves and our lives.

To be self-compassionate, mindfulness is actually the first step we need to take—we need presence of mind to respond in a new way. So immediately after the office party faux pas, for instance, instead of drowning her sorrows in a box of chocolates, Theresa summoned the courage needed to face what had happened.

Theresa added: "I just acknowledged how bad I felt in the moment. I wish it didn't happen, but it did happen. What was amazing is that I could actually be with the feelings of embarrassment, the flushed cheeks, the heat rising in my head, without getting lost in self-judgment. I knew the feelings wouldn't kill me, and they would eventually pass. And they did. I gave myself a little pep talk, saw my coworker the next day to apologize and explain myself, and everything was fine."

> Cultivating a state of loving, connected presence can change our relationship with ourselves and the world around us.

Another way to describe the three essential elements of self-compassion is *loving* (self-kindness), *connected* (common humanity) *presence* (mindfulness). When we are in the mind state of loving, connected presence, our relationship to ourselves, others, and the world is transformed.

EXERCISE
How Do I Treat a Friend?

- Close your eyes and reflect for a moment on the following question:
    - Think about various times when you've had a close friend who was struggling in some way—had a misfortune, failed, or felt inadequate—and you were feeling pretty good about yourself. How do you typically respond to your friends in such situations? What do you say? What tone do you use? How is your posture? Nonverbal gestures?

- Write down what you discovered.

. Wow that must be so hard. I can totally understand why you feel that way. You deserve so much better.

. Kind voice

- Straight back.

- Now close your eyes again and reflect on the next question:

  - Think about various times when *you* were struggling in some way—had a misfortune, failed, or felt inadequate. How do you typically respond to yourself in these situations? What do you say? What tone do you use? Your posture? Nonverbal gestures?

- Write down what you discovered.

Whats wrong w/ you? I feel so small. Why can't I manage to get anything done. whats wrong w/ me? I'm so lazy.

Slouchy

- Finally, consider the differences between how you treat your close friends when they are struggling and how you treat yourself. Do you notice any patterns?

I am much meaner to myself. I really become a different person w/ friend vs. me. I am so much clearer and more confident in the friend example. I'm so down and mean to myself, almost like a depressed person.

REFLECTION

What came up for you while doing this practice?

When they do this exercise many people are shocked at how badly they treat themselves compared to their friends. If you are one of these people, you are not alone. Preliminary data suggests that the vast majority of people are more compassionate to others than to themselves. Our culture doesn't encourage us to be kind to ourselves, so we need to intentionally practice changing our relationship with ourselves in order to counter the habits of a lifetime.

 EXERCISE

Relating to Ourselves with Self-Compassion

Think about a current struggle you're going through in your life—one that's not too serious. For example, maybe you had a fight with your partner and you said something you regret. Or maybe you really blew it on a work assignment and you're frightened your boss is going to call you in for a meeting to reprimand you.

- Write down the situation.

The mother who didn't text back

- First write down any ways you may be lost in the story line of the situation and running away with it. Is it all you can think about, or are you making a bigger deal out of things than is warranted? For example, are you terrified that you will be fired even though the mistake was pretty minor?

I thought about it a lot - a lot of ruminating. I made a lot of assumptions.

- Now see if you can mindfully acknowledge the pain involved in this situation without exaggerating it or being overly dramatic. Write down any painful or difficult feelings you may be having, trying to do so with a relatively objective and balanced tone. Validate the difficulty of the situation, while trying not to get overly caught up in the story line of what you're feeling. For example: "I'm feeling really frightened that I will get in trouble with my boss after this incident. It's difficult for me to feel this right now."

Im feeling embarassed and potentially bothered to have a false or negative view of myself.

- Next write down any ways you may be feeling isolated by the situation, thinking that it shouldn't have happened or that you're the only one who has been in this situation. For example, are you assuming that your work should be perfect and that it's abnormal to make mistakes? That no one else at your work makes these types of mistakes?

Feeling singled out in this mothers perspective (or potentially).

- Now try to remind yourself of the common humanity of the situation—how normal it is to have feelings like this and the fact that many people are probably experiencing feelings similar to yours. For example: "I guess it's natural to feel frightened after making a mistake at work. Everyone makes mistakes sometimes, and I'm sure many other people have been in a similar situation to what I'm facing right now."

Perhaps other ppl would also feel off from her lack of response & abruptness.

- Next write down any ways you may be judging yourself for what happened. For example, are you calling yourself names ("stupid idiot") or being overly harsh with yourself ("You are always messing up. Why can't you ever learn?")?

- Finally, try writing yourself some words of kindness in response to the difficult emotions you are feeling. Write using the same type of gentle, supportive words you might use with a good friend you cared about. For example: "I'm so sorry that you're feeling frightened right now. I'm sure it will be okay, and I'll be here to support you whatever happens." Or else, "It's okay to make mistakes, and it's okay to feel scared about the consequences. I know you did your best."

Its totally understandable to feel the way you did.
It must hurt to feel judged.
I will be here to support you even if the
assumptions are true and will love you for who
you are anyways. You are doing your best.

REFLECTION

What was this practice like for you? Take a moment and try to fully accept how you're feeling in this moment, allowing yourself to be just as you are.

Some people feel soothed and comforted by words of mindfulness, common humanity, and self-kindness when they do this writing exercise. If it felt supportive for you, can you allow yourself to savor the feeling of caring for yourself in this way?

For many people, however, writing in this way feels awkward or uncomfortable. If this describes your experience, can you allow yourself to learn at your own pace, knowing that it takes time to form new habits?

It felt good by the final exercise to love myself as I am and for who I am. Surprisingly.

2

What Self-Compassion Is Not

Often people have misgivings about whether it's a good idea to be self-compassionate or whether we can be *too* self-compassionate. Certainly Western culture doesn't promote self-compassion as a virtue, and many people harbor deep suspicions about being kind to themselves. These misgivings often block our ability to be self-compassionate, so it's good to take a close look at them.

EXERCISE

My Misgivings about Self-Compassion

- Write down any misgivings that you personally have about self-compassion—any fears or concerns you have about its possible downsides.

> Only that I might "miss" something I need to be aware of.

- Sometimes our attitudes are shaped by what other people in our life think about self-compassion. Write down any misgivings that other people or society at large have about self-compassion.

> Probably self-compassion in society-seen as selfish.

REFLECTION

If you identified some misgivings that you hold, that's a good thing. These misgivings are actually barriers to your ability to be self-compassionate, and awareness is the first step toward starting to dismantle these barriers.

Fortunately, an ever-increasing body of research shows that the most common misgivings about self-compassion are actually misconceptions. In other words, our misconceptions are generally unfounded. Below are some of the fears people express over and over again at our courses, followed by a brief description of the evidence to the contrary.

> *Misgivings about self-compassion are likely to be misconceptions.*

"Doesn't self-compassion just mean throwing a pity party for poor me?"

Many people fear that self-compassion is really just a form of self-pity. In fact, self-compassion is an *antidote* to self-pity. While self-pity says "poor me," self-compassion recognizes that life is hard for everyone. Research shows that self-compassionate people are more likely to engage in perspective taking, rather than focusing on their own distress. They are also *less* likely to ruminate on how bad things are, which is one of the reasons self-compassionate people have better mental health. When we are self-compassionate, we remember that everyone suffers from time to time (common humanity), and we don't exaggerate the extent of our struggles (mindfulness). Self-compassion is not a "woe is me" attitude.

"Self-compassion is for wimps. I have to be tough and strong to get through my life."

Another big fear is that self-compassion will make us weak and vulnerable. In fact, self-compassion is a reliable source of inner strength that confers courage and enhances resilience when we're faced with difficulties. Research shows self-compassionate people are better able to cope with tough situations like divorce, trauma, or chronic pain.

"I need to think more about other people, not myself. Being self-compassionate is way too selfish and self-focused."

Some worry that by being self-compassionate rather than just focusing on being compassionate to others, they will become self-centered or selfish. However, giving compassion to ourselves actually enables us to give more to others in relationships. Research shows self-compassionate people tend to be more caring and supportive in romantic relationships, are more likely to compromise in relationship conflicts, and are more compassionate and forgiving toward others.

"Self-compassion will make me lazy. I will probably just skip work whenever I feel like it and stay in bed eating chocolate chip cookies all day!"

Although many people fear that being self-compassionate means being self-indulgent, it's actually just the opposite. Compassion inclines us toward long-term health and well-being, not short-term pleasure (just as a compassionate mother doesn't let her child eat all the ice cream she wants, but says, "eat your vegetables"). Research shows self-compassionate people engage in healthier behaviors like exercise, eating well, drinking less, and going to the doctor more regularly.

"If I'm compassionate to myself, I'll let myself get away with murder. I need to be hard on myself when I mess up to make sure I don't hurt other people."

Another fear is that self-compassion is really a form of making excuses for bad behavior. Actually, self-compassion provides the safety needed to admit mistakes rather than needing to blame someone else for them. Research shows that self-compassionate people take greater personal responsibility for their actions and are more likely to apologize if they've offended someone.

"I will never get to where I want in life if I let up on my harsh self-criticism for even one moment. It's what drives me to succeed. Self-compassion is fine for some people, but I have high standards and goals I want to achieve in my life."

The most common misgiving people have is that self-compassion might undermine their motivation to achieve. Most people believe self-criticism is an effective motivator, but it's not. Self-criticism tends to undermine self-confidence and leads to fear of failure. If we are self-compassionate, we will still be motivated to reach our goals—not because we're inadequate as we are, but because we care about ourselves and want to reach our full potential (see Chapter 11). Research shows that self-compassionate people have high personal standards; they just don't beat themselves up when they fail. This means they are less afraid of failure and are more likely to try again and to persist in their efforts after failing.

MIRROR, MIRROR ON THE WALL

Often when telling people about self-compassion, we get this type of comment.

"That's just like Stuart Smalley on *Saturday Night Live,* who loved to gaze in the mirror and say 'I'm good enough, I'm smart enough, and doggone it, people like me!' Isn't it?"

To truly understand what self-compassion is, it's important to distinguish it from a close cousin—self-esteem. In Western culture, high self-esteem requires standing out in a crowd—being special and above average. The problem, of course, is that it's impossible for *everyone* to be above average at the same time. While there may be some areas in which we excel, there's always someone more attractive, success-ful, and intelligent than we are, meaning we feel like failures whenever we compare ourselves to those "bet-ter" than ourselves.

> *Self-compassion should not be confused with self-esteem.*

The desire to see ourselves as better than average, however, and to *keep* that elusive feeling of high self-esteem, can lead to some downright nasty behavior. Why do early adolescents begin to bully others? If I can be seen as the cool tough kid in contrast to the wimpy nerd I just picked on, I get a self-esteem boost. Why are we so prejudiced? If I believe that my ethnic, gender, national, or political group is better than yours, I get a self-esteem boost.

But self-compassion is different from self-esteem. Although they're both strongly linked to psychological well-being, they diverge in significant ways:

- Self-esteem is a positive evaluation of self-worth. Self-compassion isn't a judgment or an evaluation at all. Instead, self-compassion is way of *relating* to the ever-changing landscape of who we are with kindness and acceptance—especially when we fail or feel inadequate.

- Self-esteem requires feeling better than others. Self-compassion requires acknowledging that we are all imperfect.

- Self-esteem tends to be a fair-weather friend, there for us when we succeed but deserting us precisely when we need it the most—when we fail or make a fool of ourselves. Self-compassion is always there for us, a reliable source of support even when our worldly stock has crashed. It still hurts when our pride is dashed, but we can be kind to ourselves *because* it hurts. "Wow, that was pretty humiliating. I'm so sorry. It's okay though; these things happen."

- Compared with self-esteem, self-compassion is less contingent on conditions like physical attractiveness or successful performance and provides a more stable sense of self-worth over time. It is also linked to less social comparison and narcissism than self-esteem is.

EXERCISE
How Is Self-Esteem Working for You?

- How do you feel when you receive the feedback that your performance is average in an area of life that you care about (e.g., work, parenting, friend-ship, romance)?

I don't know if I've received that, but I would feel really low.

- How do you feel when someone is *better* at doing something you really care about (e.g., achieving more sales, baking tastier cookies for the school party, being a better basketball player, looking better in a swimsuit)? I

think its hard to determine better. But also I'm used to it. I feel I normally see people as being better, but I want to be the "best" or top. Or sometimes I think - I could do it better.

- How does it impact you when you *fail* at something that you care about (e.g., your teaching evaluations are poor, your kid says you're a horrible dad, you don't get asked out for a second date)? I think I should give up, or not for me, I'll find something I'm better at.

REFLECTION

If you're like most people, you'll find that it doesn't feel okay to be average, that you don't like it when people outperform you, and that—to put it bluntly— failure sucks. This is only human. But it's important to consider that these are all major limitations of self-esteem: self-esteem causes us to constantly compare ourselves to others and means that our self-worth bounces up and down like a Ping-Pong ball depending on our latest success or failure. When we notice that our need for high self-esteem is causing problems for us, it's time to practice a new way of relating to ourselves—with self-compassion!

I have a need for high self-esteem?
I have a need for being seen for what I can contribute. That people see me as a mentor, leader, someone to look to for answers and advice and guidance. To be someone who creates. I feel incomplete without those 2 things: being a "guider" and a "creator." So what then? Stop wanting that? Love myself without it? Find ways I already do it?

3

The Benefits of Self-Compassion

On the first night of our course, Marion was pretty skeptical. "How will self-compassion help me? I'm in the habit of being really hard on myself— it's the devil I know. It's what got me to where I am today. Why should I change? Can I change? How can I be sure it's a safe thing to do?"

Luckily, Marion didn't have to just take our word for it. Over a thousand research studies have demonstrated the mental and physical health benefits of self-compassion.

People who are more self-compassionate experience greater well-being:

Less	More
Depression	Happiness
Anxiety	Life satisfaction
Stress	Self-confidence
Shame	Physical health

Although people naturally vary in terms of how self-compassionate they are, it is also the case that self-compassion can be learned. Research has shown that people who took the MSC course (the program this workbook is based on) increased their levels of self-compassion by an average of 43%. Participation in the course also helped them to become more mindful and compassionate toward others, feel more social connectedness, life satisfaction, and happiness, and be less depressed, anxious, and stressed. Participants were also less likely to avoid their difficult emotions after taking MSC.

Most of these benefits were tied directly to learning to be more self-compassionate. Moreover, the increase in self-compassion and other benefits of MSC were maintained one year later. Gains in self-compassion were linked to how much self-compassion

Almost never				Almost always
1	2	3	4	5

_____ I try to see my failings as part of the human condition.

_____ When I'm going through a very hard time, I give myself the caring and tenderness I need.

_____ When something upsets me, I try to keep my emotions in balance.

_____ When I feel inadequate in some way, I try to remind myself that feelings of inadequacy are shared by most people.

For the next set of items, use the following scale (notice that the endpoints of the scale are reversed from those above):

Almost always				Almost never
1	2	3	4	5

_____ When I fail at something important to me, I become consumed by feelings of inadequacy.

_____ When I'm feeling down, I tend to feel like most other people are probably happier than I am.

_____ When I fail at something that's important to me, I tend to feel alone in my failure.

_____ When I'm feeling down, I tend to obsess and fixate on everything that's wrong.

_____ I'm disapproving and judgmental about my own flaws and inadequacies.

_____ I'm intolerant and impatient toward those aspects of my personality I don't like.

How to score your test:

Total (sum of all 12 items)   _____

Mean score = Total/12   _____

Average overall self-compassion scores tend to be around 3.0 on the 1–5 scale, so you can interpret your overall score accordingly. As a rough guide, a score of 1–2.5 for your overall self-compassion score indicates you are low in self-compassion, 2.5–3.5 indicates you are moderate, and 3.5–5.0 means you are high in self-compassion.

REFLECTION

If you scored lower in self-compassion than you would like, don't worry. The beautiful thing about self-compassion is that it is a skill that can be learned. You might just have to give yourself some time, but it will happen eventually.

INFORMAL PRACTICE
Keeping a Self-Compassion Journal

Try writing a self-compassion journal every day for one week (or longer if you like). Journaling is an effective way to express emotions and has been found to enhance both mental and physical well-being.

At some point during the evening, when you have a few quiet moments, review the day's events. In your journal, write down anything that you felt bad about, anything you judged yourself for, or any difficult experience that caused you pain. (For instance, perhaps you got angry at the waitstaff at a restaurant because they took forever to bring the check. You made a rude comment and stormed off without leaving a tip. Afterward, you felt ashamed and embarrassed.) For each difficult event that happened during the day, try mindfulness, a sense of common humanity, and kindness to relate to the event in a more self-compassionate way. Here's how:

Mindfulness

This will mainly involve bringing balanced awareness to the painful emotions that arose due to your self-judgment or difficult circumstances. Write about how you felt: sad, ashamed, frightened, stressed, and so on. As you write, try to be accepting and nonjudgmental of your experience, without diminishing it or becoming overly dramatic. (For example, "I was frustrated because the waitperson was so slow. I got angry, overreacted, and felt foolish afterward.")

Common Humanity

Write down the ways in which your experience was part of being human. This might include acknowledging that being human means being imperfect and that all people have these sorts of painful experiences. ("Everyone overreacts sometimes—it's only human." "This is how people are likely to feel in a situation like that.") You might also want to think about the unique causes and conditions underlying your painful event. ("My frustration was exacerbated by the fact that I was half an hour late for my doctor's appointment across town and there was a lot of traffic that day. If the circumstances had been different, my reaction probably would have been different.")

Self-Kindness

Write yourself some kind, understanding words, much as you might write to a good friend. Let yourself know that you care about your happiness and well-being, adopting a gentle, reassuring tone. ("It's okay. You messed up, but it wasn't the end of the world. I understand how frustrated you were and you just lost it. Maybe you can try being extra patient and generous to any waitstaff you encounter this week.")

REFLECTION

After keeping your self-compassion journal for at least a week, ask yourself if you noticed any changes in your internal dialogue. How did it feel to write to yourself in a more self-compassionate manner? Do you think it helped you to cope with the difficulties that arose?

Some people will find that keeping a self-compassion journal is a wonderful way to help support their practice, while for others it may seem like a chore. It's probably worth trying it out for a week or so, but if journal writing isn't your thing, you can skip the writing part. The important thing is that we practice all three steps of self-compassion—mindfully turning toward our pain, remembering that imperfection is part of the shared human experience, and being kind and supportive to ourselves because things are difficult.

4

The Physiology of Self-Criticism and Self-Compassion

According to Paul Gilbert, who created compassion-focused therapy (CFT), when we criticize ourselves we're tapping into the body's threat-defense system (sometimes referred to as our reptilian brain). Among the many ways we can react to perceived danger, the threat-defense system is the quickest and most easily triggered. This means that self-criticism is often our first reaction when things go wrong.

The threat-defense system evolved so that when we perceive a threat, our amygdala (which registers danger in the brain) gets activated, we release cortisol and adrenaline, and we get ready to fight, flee, or freeze. The system works well for protecting against threats to our physical bodies, but nowadays most of the threats we face are challenges to our self-image or self-concept.

Feeling threatened puts stress on the mind and body, and chronic stress can cause anxiety and depression, which is why habitual self-criticism is so bad for emotional and physical well-being. With self-criticism, we are both the attacker and the attacked.

> *When we feel inadequate, our self-concept is threatened, so we attack the problem—ourselves!*

Luckily, we're not just reptiles, but also mammals. The evolutionary advance of mammals is that mammalian young are born very immature and have a longer developmental period to adapt to their environment. To keep infants safe during this vulnerable period, the mammalian care system evolved, prompting parents and offspring to stay close.

When the care system is activated, oxytocin (the love hormone) and endorphins (natural feel-good opiates) are released, which helps reduce stress and increase feelings of safety and security. Two reliable ways of activating the care system are soothing touch and gentle vocalizations (think of a cat purring and licking her kittens).

REFLECTION

Take a moment to reflect on how the experience of this exercise was for you. Did you notice anything after you evoked mindfulness with the first phrase, "This is a moment of suffering"? Any shifts?

How about the second phrase, reminding you of common humanity, or the third, which invited self-kindness? Were you able to find kindhearted words you would say to a friend, and if so, what was it like to say the same words to yourself? Easy? More difficult?

Sometimes it takes a bit of time to find language that works for you personally and feels authentic. Allow yourself to be a slow learner—eventually you will find the right words.

Note that this informal practice can be done slowly as a sort of mini-meditation, or you can use the words as a three-part mantra when you encounter difficulties in daily life.

 INFORMAL PRACTICE

Compassionate Movement

This informal practice can be used whenever you need a stretch break. It can be practiced with open or closed eyes. The main idea is to move compassionately from the inside out, not necessarily in prescribed ways.

Anchoring

- Stand up and feel the soles of your feet on the floor. Rock forward and backward a little and side to side. Make little circles with your knees, feeling the changes of sensation in the soles of your feet. Anchor your awareness in your feet.

Opening

- Now open your field of awareness and scan your whole body for other sensations, noticing any areas of ease as well as areas of tension.

Responding Compassionately

- Now focus for a moment on any places of *discomfort*.
    - Gradually begin to move your body in a way that feels really good to you—giving yourself compassion. For example, let yourself gently twist your shoulders, roll your head, turn at the waist, drop into a forward bend . . . whatever feels just right for you now.
    - Give your body the movement it needs, letting your body guide you.
    - Sometimes our bodies disappoint us, or we're not happy with the way

4

The Physiology of Self-Criticism and Self-Compassion

According to Paul Gilbert, who created compassion-focused therapy (CFT), when we criticize ourselves we're tapping into the body's threat-defense system (sometimes referred to as our reptilian brain). Among the many ways we can react to perceived danger, the threat-defense system is the quickest and most easily triggered. This means that self-criticism is often our first reaction when things go wrong.

The threat-defense system evolved so that when we perceive a threat, our amygdala (which registers danger in the brain) gets activated, we release cortisol and adrenaline, and we get ready to fight, flee, or freeze. The system works well for protecting against threats to our physical bodies, but nowadays most of the threats we face are challenges to our self-image or self-concept.

> *When we feel inadequate, our self-concept is threatened, so we attack the problem—ourselves!*

Feeling threatened puts stress on the mind and body, and chronic stress can cause anxiety and depression, which is why habitual self-criticism is so bad for emotional and physical well-being. With self-criticism, we are both the attacker and the attacked.

Luckily, we're not just reptiles, but also mammals. The evolutionary advance of mammals is that mammalian young are born very immature and have a longer developmental period to adapt to their environment. To keep infants safe during this vulnerable period, the mammalian care system evolved, prompting parents and offspring to stay close.

When the care system is activated, oxytocin (the love hormone) and endorphins (natural feel-good opiates) are released, which helps reduce stress and increase feelings of safety and security. Two reliable ways of activating the care system are soothing touch and gentle vocalizations (think of a cat purring and licking her kittens).

Compassion, including *self*-compassion, is linked to the mammalian care system. That's why being compassionate to ourselves when we feel inadequate makes us feel safe and cared for, like a child held in a warm embrace.

> *Extending compassion to ourselves when we feel insecure is like getting comfort from a parent.*

Self-compassion helps to downregulate the threat response. When the stress response (fight–flight–freeze) is triggered by a threat to our self-concept, we are likely to turn on ourselves in an unholy trinity of reactions. We fight ourselves (self-criticism), we flee from others (isolation), or we freeze (rumination). These three reactions are precisely the opposite of the three components of self-compassion—self-kindness, common humanity, and mindfulness. The following table illustrates the relationship of the stress response to self-compassion.

Stress Response	Stress Response Turned Inward	Self-Compassion
Fight	Self-criticism	Self-kindness
Flight	Isolation	Common humanity
Freeze	Rumination	Mindfulness

When we practice self-compassion, we are deactivating the threat-defense system and activating the care system. In one study, for instance, researchers asked participants to imagine receiving compassion and feeling it in their bodies. Every minute they were told things like "Allow yourself to feel that you are the recipient of great compassion; allow yourself to feel the loving-kindness that is there for you." It was found that the participants given these instructions had lower cortisol levels after the imagery than those in the control group. Participants also demonstrated increased heart-rate variability afterward. The safer people feel, the more open and flexible they can be in response to their environment, and this is reflected in how much their heart rate varies in response to stimuli. So you could say that when they gave themselves compassion, participants' hearts actually opened and became less defensive.

Thomas was a good, conscientious man who volunteered at his church and could always be counted on to lend a helping hand to others. He was also a relentless self-critic. He criticized himself for almost everything—he wasn't successful enough, smart enough, giving enough. He was too self-critical! Whenever Thomas noticed anything he did that he didn't like about himself, the insults began. "Lame-ass. Stupid fool. Loser." Constant self-criticism was wearing him down, and he started to become depressed.

After learning that self-criticism is associated with feeling threatened, Thomas wondered what he might be afraid of that made him so self-critical. It immediately became clear to him that he was afraid of being rejected. As a

child, Thomas was badly bullied for having learning differences and never felt he fit in. There was a part of him that believed that if he bullied and attacked himself for his inadequacies now, it would somehow miraculously motivate him to do better so that others would accept him while also protecting him from the pain of being judged—he'd beat them to the punch. Of course, self-criticism didn't work—it just made him depressed.

Thomas had also learned that he could feel safe by activating the care system—simple things like speaking to himself in a friendly, understanding way. So he gave it a try. When the slew of insults began, he would catch himself: "I see you feel afraid and you're trying to protect yourself." Eventually he started to add things like "It's okay. You aren't perfect, but you're trying your best." Although the habit of self-criticism was still strong, acknowledging where it came from helped him to not get so sucked into it and gave him hope that, with time, he could learn to treat himself with the kindness and acceptance he wasn't shown as a child.

 INFORMAL PRACTICE
Soothing Touch

Although it may seem a bit "touchy-feely" at first—and in fact it is—it's useful to harness the power of physical touch to help us trigger the compassion response. By putting one or two hands on our physical body in a warm, caring, and gentle way, we can help ourselves to feel safe and comforted. It's important to note that different physical gestures evoke different emotional responses in different people. The invitation is to find a manner of physical touch that feels genuinely supportive, so that you can use this gesture to care for yourself whenever you're under stress.

> *What touch do I need to feel safe and comforted?*

Find a private space where you don't have to worry about anyone watching you. Below is a list of different ways that people comfort themselves with touch. Go ahead and try them out, and also feel free to experiment on your own. You may want to do this exploration with your eyes closed so you can focus on what feels just right for you.

- ✧ One hand over your heart
- ✧ Two hands over your heart
- ✧ Gently stroking your chest
- ✧ Cupping your hand over a fist over your heart
- ✧ One hand on your heart and one on your belly
- ✧ Two hands on your belly
- ✧ One hand on your cheek

✧ Cradling your face in your hands

✧ Gently stroking your arms

✧ Crossing your arms and giving yourself a gentle hug

✧ One hand tenderly holding the other

✧ Cupping your hands in your lap

Continue your exploration until you find a type of touch that is truly comforting—everyone is different.

REFLECTION

What was this practice like for you? Were you able to find a gesture that felt genuinely soothing and supportive?

If you found a physical touch that works for you, try adopting this gesture whenever you feel stress or emotional pain in everyday life. By helping your body feel cared for and safe, you will make it easier for your mind and heart to follow.

Sometimes it can feel awkward or uncomfortable when we give ourselves soothing touch, however. In fact, "backdraft" often arises—a concept we will discuss further in Chapter 8. *Backdraft* refers to old pains that emerge when we give ourselves kindness, such as remembering times when we were *not* treated kindly. This is why soothing touch might not feel soothing. If that happens to you, you can try touching an external object that is warm and soft, like petting a dog or cat, or holding a pillow. Or maybe a firmer gesture would feel better, such as tapping or fist-bumping your own chest. The point is to express care and kindness in a manner that meets your own needs.

INFORMAL PRACTICE
Self-Compassion Break

This practice is a way to help remind ourselves to apply the three core components of self-compassion—mindfulness, common humanity, and kindness—when difficulties arise in our lives. It also harnesses the power of soothing touch to help us feel safe and cared for. It's important to find language that is effective for you personally—you don't want to have an internal argument about whether the words make sense. For example, some people prefer the word *struggle* to the word *suffering,* or prefer the word *support* or *protect* to the word *kindness.* Try out a few different variations and then practice what works for you.

After reading through these instructions, you may want to try them out with your eyes closed so you can go inward more deeply. You can also find a guided recording of this practice online (see the end of the Contents for information).

- Think of a situation in your life that is causing you stress, such as a health problem, relationship problem, work problem, or some other struggle.

  Choose a problem in the mild to moderate range, not a big problem, as we want to build the resource of self-compassion gradually.

- Visualize the situation clearly in your mind's eye. What is the setting? Who is saying what to whom? What is happening? What *might* happen?

  Can you feel discomfort in your body as you bring this difficulty to mind? If not, choose a slightly more difficult problem.

- Now, try saying to yourself: "This is a moment of suffering."

  o That's mindfulness. Perhaps other wording speaks to you better. Some options are:

    • *This hurts.*
    • *Ouch.*
    • *This is stressful.*

- Now, try saying to yourself: "Suffering is a part of life."

  o That's common humanity. Other options include:

    • *I'm not alone.*
    • *Everyone experiences this, just like me.*
    • *This is how it feels when people struggle in this way.*

- Now, offer yourself the gesture of soothing touch that you discovered in the previous exercise.

- And try saying to yourself: "May I be kind to myself" or "May I give myself what I need."

  Perhaps there are particular words of kindness and support that you need to hear right now in this difficult situation. Some options may be:

  o *May I accept myself as I am.*
  o *May I begin to accept myself as I am.*
  o *May I forgive myself.*
  o *May I be strong.*
  o *May I be patient.*

- If you're having difficulty finding the right words, imagine that a dear friend or loved one is having the same problem as you. What would you say to this person? What simple message would you like to deliver to your friend, heart to heart?

  Now see if you can offer the same message to yourself.

REFLECTION

Take a moment to reflect on how the experience of this exercise was for you. Did you notice anything after you evoked mindfulness with the first phrase, "This is a moment of suffering"? Any shifts?

How about the second phrase, reminding you of common humanity, or the third, which invited self-kindness? Were you able to find kindhearted words you would say to a friend, and if so, what was it like to say the same words to yourself? Easy? More difficult?

Sometimes it takes a bit of time to find language that works for you personally and feels authentic. Allow yourself to be a slow learner—eventually you will find the right words.

Note that this informal practice can be done slowly as a sort of mini-meditation, or you can use the words as a three-part mantra when you encounter difficulties in daily life.

 INFORMAL PRACTICE
Compassionate Movement

This informal practice can be used whenever you need a stretch break. It can be practiced with open or closed eyes. The main idea is to move compassionately from the inside out, not necessarily in prescribed ways.

Anchoring

- Stand up and feel the soles of your feet on the floor. Rock forward and backward a little and side to side. Make little circles with your knees, feeling the changes of sensation in the soles of your feet. Anchor your awareness in your feet.

Opening

- Now open your field of awareness and scan your whole body for other sensations, noticing any areas of ease as well as areas of tension.

Responding Compassionately

- Now focus for a moment on any places of *discomfort*.
    - Gradually begin to move your body in a way that feels really good to you—giving yourself compassion. For example, let yourself gently twist your shoulders, roll your head, turn at the waist, drop into a forward bend . . . whatever feels just right for you now.
    - Give your body the movement it needs, letting your body guide you.
    - Sometimes our bodies disappoint us, or we're not happy with the way

they look or feel or move. If that is so for you, just be with yourself and your tender heart for a moment. Your body is doing its best. What do you need right now?

Coming to Stillness

- Finally, come to stillness. Stand again and feel your entire body, noting any changes.
  - Allow yourself to be just as you are in this moment.

REFLECTION

Take a moment to reflect on how the experience of this exercise was for you. Did it feel different to stretch as an intentional caring response to discomfort? Were you able to find a way of moving that gave your body what it needed?

This practice can be used multiple times throughout the day. Whether or not your body feels better after stretching is actually less important than the intention to notice where you're holding tension in your body and responding in a caring manner. We often ignore our bodies' subtle distress signals, and getting into the habit of checking in and intentionally giving ourselves what we need can go a long way toward developing a healthier and more supportive self-to-self relationship.

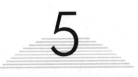

5

The Yin and Yang
of Self-Compassion

At first glance, compassion may seem like a soft quality, associated only with comforting and soothing. Because compassion for others is a part of nurturing, especially caring for children, we may also instinctively link it to more traditional feminine gender role norms. Does this mean self-compassion isn't really for all of us? Ask yourself this: Is it any less compassionate to enter a burning building to rescue a person trapped inside or to work long hours to provide for a family—behaviors linked to more masculine and action-oriented gender-role norms and hardly characterized as soft? We clearly need to expand our cultural understanding of compassion and self-compassion to make room for its many manifestations.

When we explore the attributes that are at play in self-compassion, we find both the feminine and the masculine—just as all people embody both feminine and masculine qualities. In traditional Chinese philosophy, this duality is represented by *yin* and *yang*. Yin and yang are based on the assumption that all seemingly opposite attributes, such as male–female, light–dark, and active–passive, are complementary and interdependent. This means that people who identify as male or female need their opposite qualities to be in balance. Significantly, each side of the yin–yang symbol has a dot of the opposite color contained within it.

- The *yin* of self-compassion contains the attributes of "being with" ourselves in a compassionate way—*comforting, soothing, validating* ourselves.

- The *yang* of self-compassion is about "acting in the world"—*protecting, providing,* and *motivating* ourselves.

Monique wasn't so sure about self-compassion. She grew up in a rough neighborhood and would proudly tell anyone who'd listen how she survived by developing grit and street smarts at an early age. Whenever she faced a challenge, she would go at it head-on, without hesitating. She also recently received a diagnosis of multiple sclerosis, for which her usual approach to solving problems wasn't so helpful. Monique's family, friends, and even her doctors had to endure a tongue-lashing from Monique whenever she felt vulnerable and afraid about her diagnosis and the prescribed course of rest and relaxation. Frantic activity usually protected Monique against facing her emotions, but it was a poor defense against MS. And the whole self-compassion idea of being gentle and kind to yourself was anathema to Monique, who considered herself tough and stoic.

Xavier had the opposite problem. Although his childhood also wasn't easy and his stepfather was always shouting at his mother, he learned to take refuge in his books, being as unobtrusive as possible until the domestic storms passed. Xavier realized at an early age that confrontation would only make things worse. Now Xavier was in his early 20s, his college years were behind him, and he needed to get on with his life, starting with earning enough money to get out of his mother's basement. However, Xavier wasn't sure he could do it. He took a job as an orderly at a hospital, just to get out of the house, but remained deeply unsatisfied. Xavier needed someone to believe in him and also to encourage him to achieve what he was capable of.

MSC contains a wide variety of practices and exercises that each person can explore to discover which ones work best. Some practices fit more into the yin category and some into the yang category, although most have aspects of both. The table below gives examples of practices in this book that generally correspond to the yin or yang attributes of self-compassion. Of course, these attributes themselves interact and are interdependent. For example, when we validate our needs, we often find the motivation to fulfill them in our lives.

Cultivating the Yin and Yang of Self-Compassion

	Attributes	Practices
	Comforting	Self-Compassion Break (Ch. 4) Self-Compassion in Daily Life (Ch. 8) Loving-Kindness for Ourselves Meditation (Ch. 10)
Yin	Soothing	Soothing Touch (Ch. 4) Affectionate Breathing Meditation (Ch. 6) Soften–Soothe–Allow (Ch. 16)
	Validating	Being a Compassionate Mess (Ch. 13) Labeling Emotions (Ch. 16) Self-Appreciation (Ch. 23)

Attributes	Practices
Protecting	Feeling the Soles of Your Feet (Ch. 8) Compassion with Equanimity (Ch. 19) Fierce Compassion (Ch. 20)
Providing	Discovering Our Core Values (Ch. 14) Fulfilling Our Emotional Needs (Ch. 18) Meeting Unmet Needs (Ch. 20)
Motivating	Finding Your Compassionate Voice (Ch. 11) Compassionate Letter to Myself (Ch. 11) Living with a Vow (Ch. 14)

Yang

A common thread through all these practices is a friendly, caring attitude. Sometimes self-compassionate care takes the form of solace and a soft leaning in to difficult emotions (comforting), sometimes it involves a stern "no!" and turning away from danger (protecting). Sometimes it involves letting our bodies know everything is okay with warmth and tenderness (soothing), and sometimes it means figuring out what we need and giving it to ourselves (providing). Sometimes self-compassion requires being accepting and open to what is (validating), and sometimes it means we need to jump up and do something about it (motivating).

Monique was adept at the yang qualities of strength, action, and determination for meeting challenges to her safety and well-being. She knew how to protect and provide for herself. Her yin, more receptive side was relatively underdeveloped, perhaps because it wasn't safe for her to be receptive and validating of "what is" as a child. Monique's MS diagnosis meant she needed to learn new skills to get her through. Monique's friend told her about the Self-Compassion Break (Chapter 4), which is a combination of different elements of self-compassion, but especially the attributes of validating her situation ("it's so scary to get an MS diagnosis"), realizing she's not alone ("having a major illness makes almost everyone feel vulnerable and alone"), and then offering herself words of comfort: "It's going to be okay. Let's take this one day at a time." The Self-Compassion Break opened the door to self-compassion for Monique. It wasn't an easy road for her, however, due to lots of old pain in early relationships when she was young and vulnerable. But Monique had the gift of courage, and MS had a silver lining—because she had to accept her condition, Monique began to experience an inner peace of acceptance that she didn't know was possible.

Xavier, on the other hand, didn't have a lot of drive, but he had a tender heart. His drive was squelched by his angry stepfather, who always had to have the last word, and he became adept at avoiding conflict by staying in the shadows. Now he needed strength and courage, however, to step out into the world. Quite by accident, Xavier saw a flyer at his hospital about a brief self-compassion training for healthcare workers. In this course, Xavier discovered that the same inner voice that told him to stay safe by staying invisible at home was now asking him to step out. The best self-compassion practice for Xavier was writing a compassionate letter (Chapter 11) to motivate himself with kindness, just as he might write to a dear friend in a similar situation. He wrote himself a letter every week, focusing on whatever challenges he encountered. Little by little, a new voice emerged within Xavier—his own inner coach cheering him on from the sidelines. Over time, Xavier was able to claim what he needed for a meaningful life—his core values—and he took practical steps to actualize them in his life.

EXERCISE

What Aspects of Self-Compassion Do I Need Now?

Self-compassion probably has more different aspects than you originally thought. Some yin and yang attributes of self-compassion are listed below. Look them over and consider which attributes you might need to draw on the most right now. This will help you understand how self-compassion could be helpful as you go through this book.

Yin

- *Comforting.* Comforting is something that we might do for a dear friend who is struggling. It refers to helping a suffering person feel better, especially by providing support for his *emotional* needs. Is this something you need right now? Do you feel it would help to learn how to comfort yourself more when you are upset?

    Yes, I am very hard on myself.

- *Soothing.* Soothing is also a way to help a person feel better, and it refers particularly to helping a person feel *physically* calmer. Is this something you need more of? Would you like to feel more comfortable and relaxed in your body?

- *Validating.* We can also help a person feel better by understanding very clearly what she is going through and saying it in a kind and tender way. Do you feel alone or misunderstood and need this kind of validation? Do you think it would help to learn to validate your own feelings?

Yang

- *Protecting.* The first step toward self-compassion is feeling safe from harm. Protecting means saying no to others who are hurting us or to the harm we inflict on ourselves, often in unconscious ways. Is there some way that you are being harmed, and would you like to find the inner strength to stop it?

- *Providing.* Providing means giving ourselves what we really need. First we have to *know* what we need, then we need the conviction that we *deserve* to get our needs met, and then we have to go ahead and try to meet our needs. No one can do this for us as well as we can do it for ourselves. Would you like to learn to provide for your own needs more effectively?

- *Motivating.* Most of us have dreams and aspirations that we would like to realize in this lifetime. We also have smaller, short-term goals. Self-compassion
  motivates like a good coach, with kindness, support, and understanding, not
  harsh criticism. Do you think it would be helpful to learn to motivate yourself
  with love instead of fear?

REFLECTION

Hopefully, the question "What do I need now?" will arise in your mind con-
tinuously as you work your way through this book. By simply asking the question, you allow yourself a moment of self-compassion, even if you can't find an
answer or don't have the ability to meet your needs at the time.

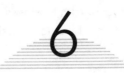

6

Mindfulness

Mindfulness is the foundation of self-compassion. We need to step outside of the story line of our suffering and turn toward our pain mindfully before we can respond with kindness. Mindfulness can be defined as "awareness of present-moment experience with acceptance." No definition adequately captures the nature of mindfulness, however, because mindfulness involves preconceptual awareness. In other words, when we are mindful we experience the world directly, not just through the lens of thought.

> *We can't respond with compassion to our own suffering until we turn toward it with mindfulness.*

Thoughts are representations—symbols that stand for reality, not reality itself. You can't smell, taste, or eat the word *apple*. When we drop below the level of thought and make direct contact with experience, we are able to get in touch with the ever-changing nature of reality. We can drop the idea of what we think reality "should" be like and open to what is. This means that when we're suffering, we can let go of the story of what is happening and simply "be" with it, and with ourselves, with courage and presence.

Terrell raised his hand and started talking about what came up for him when he practiced mindfulness at home. "My cat had to be put down recently, and I was heartbroken. My partner, Lamar, and I got that cat 12 years ago—he was like our beloved child. After getting back from the vet's office I was feeling overwhelmed, but I remembered the instructions to acknowledge the suffering and just try to be aware of what was happening in my body. I told myself 'This is so hard right now.' I felt a deep pain in my belly, like I'd just been kicked. The sense of grief was almost overwhelming. But I tried to just stay with the sensations. In fact I still feel it now, but I'm not engulfed in the pain. It's bearable."

In many ways mindfulness is a simple skill, because it just requires noticing what's happening while it's happening, using all five senses. For instance, take a moment to try focusing on what comes through the door of each of your senses, one by one.

✧ *Hearing*—Close your eyes and take a moment to listen to the sounds in the environment. Let the sounds come to you. Notice what you hear, one sound after another, with an inner nod of recognition. There is no need to name what you hear.

✧ *Sight*—Open your eyes and allow your eyes to have a soft, wide-angle gaze. Again, note whatever you see, one visual impression after the other.

✧ *Touch*—Close your eyes again and notice the sensation of touch where your body meets the chair, or your feet touch the floor.

✧ *Smell*—Put your hand up to your nose and notice any scents arising from your skin.

✧ *Taste*—Notice if there are any tastes in your mouth right now, perhaps lingering from the last thing you ate or drank.

While it's easy to be mindful for a moment or two, it is difficult to *maintain* that state of mind, because it goes against other natural tendencies of the brain. Neuroscientists have identified an interconnected network of brain regions that is active when the mind is at rest and inactive when the mind is engaged in a task—*the default mode network*. The default mode network includes structures located right down the midline of the brain, from front to back. Those parts become highly active when nothing in particular is capturing our attention, so the mind wanders.

The default mode network does three basic things: it (1) creates a sense of self, (2) projects that self into the past or the future, and (3) looks for problems. For instance, have you ever had the experience of sitting down to eat a meal, and before you knew it the entire plate of food was gone? Where was your mind? While your body was eating, your mind was elsewhere—lost in the default mode network. The brain uses its "spare" time to focus on potential problems that need solving. This is beneficial from an evolutionary point of view so that we can anticipate threats to our survival, but it's a rather unpleasant way to live.

Generally speaking, we are hardwired for survival, not for happiness.

When we're operating in the default mode, we are often struggling, but we don't have the presence of mind to *know* that we are struggling. When we are mindful, we become aware of our internal narrative and don't get so lost in it. An oft-used analogy is being at a movie theater and being swept up in the drama, clutching the armrest as the hero is about to be pushed off a cliff. Suddenly the person next to you sneezes and you realize, "Oh, that's right, I'm watching a movie!"

Mindfulness gives us mental space, and with mental space comes the freedom to choose how we might like to *respond* to a situation. Mindfulness is especially important for self-compassion training because when we suffer, mindfulness opens the door to compassion. For example, we can ask ourselves, "What do I need right now?" and try to comfort and support ourselves as we would a good friend.

Research shows that one of the benefits of practicing mindfulness regularly is that it tends to deactivate the default mode network, both while meditating and during our normal activities. This means that the more we practice being mindful, the more opportunities we have to make better choices for ourselves, including the choice to practice self-compassion.

MEDITATION
Affectionate Breathing

The following meditation trains the mind to be more focused and calm. It is a common form of mindfulness meditation—breath meditation—with added suggestions that bring affection to the process. (A guided recording of this meditation is available online; see the end of the Contents for information.)

Most of the meditation instructions in this book involve closing your eyes, but of course it's a bit hard to read with your eyes closed. Therefore, if you are not using a guided recording, you may want to read the instructions a few times before practicing the meditation, or else just open your eyes to read, close your eyes to do a few minutes of practice, then open your eyes to read again. Whatever your approach, try to make your meditation practice as lighthearted as possible, remembering that it doesn't have to be perfect (especially when the goal is self-compassion!).

- Find a posture in which your body is comfortable and will feel supported for the length of the meditation. Then let your eyes gently close, partially or fully. Take a few slow, easy breaths, releasing any unnecessary tension in your body.

- If you like, try placing a hand over your heart or another soothing place as a reminder that we're bringing not only awareness, but *affectionate* awareness, to our breathing and to ourselves. You can leave your hand there or put it back down at any time.

- Begin to notice your breathing in your body, feeling your body breathe in and feeling your body breathe out.

- Notice how your body is nourished on the inbreath and relaxes with the outbreath.

- See if you can just let your body *breathe you*. There is nothing you need to do.

- Now start to notice the *rhythm* of your breathing, flowing in and flowing out. Take some time to *feel* the natural rhythm of your breathing.

- Feel your *whole body* subtly moving with the breath, like the movement of the sea.

- Your mind will naturally wander like a curious child or a little puppy. When that happens, just gently return to the rhythm of your breathing.

- Allow your whole body to be gently rocked and caressed—*internally caressed*—by your breathing.

- If it feels right, you can *give yourself* over to your breathing, letting your breathing be all there is. Just breathing. *Being* breathing.

- And now, gently release your attention on your breath, sitting quietly in your own experience, and allow yourself to feel whatever you're feeling and to be just as you are.

- Slowly and gently open your eyes.

REFLECTION

Take a moment to reflect on what you just experienced: "What did I notice?" "What did I feel?" "How am I feeling now?"

If you were familiar with breath meditation, how was it to bring affection and appreciation into the practice, to allow yourself to be soothed by your own breath?

Did you notice that your attention increased when you *enjoyed* the breath?

Was there a difference between *being* the breath and trying to focus on the breath?

You may have noticed that your mind wandered a lot during the meditation. All minds do that—it's the default mode network in action. Please don't judge yourself for having a human mind that wanders a lot, and if you *do* judge yourself, perhaps offer yourself some compassion for that human tendency as well.

Sometimes when people do breath meditation they focus on the sensation of the breath in a particular place, as it enters and exits the nostrils, for instance, which for some causes constriction in the mind. If you noticed this happened for you, see if you can focus more on the movement of your body as it breathes. In other words, concentrate more on the gentle rocking motion created by breathing rather than focusing on the breath itself.

This is one of three core meditations in the MSC course, so you may want to try it out for about 20 minutes for a few days in a row, until you get the hang of it. If it helps to soothe and calm you, it can become part of a regular meditation practice. Remember that we recommend you do some combination of formal (meditation) and informal (daily life) practice for about 30 minutes per day.

INFORMAL PRACTICE

Here-and-Now Stone

Find a small stone that you find especially attractive. Then try the following exercise:

- Start by carefully examining your stone. Notice the colors, the angles, and the way the light plays on the surface of your stone. Allow yourself to enjoy the sight of the stone.

- Now, explore the stone with your sense of touch. Is it smooth or rough? What is its temperature?

- Let yourself become absorbed in your stone, pouring yourself into the experience of handling this beautiful stone.

- Allow yourself to experience your stone with all your senses, appreciating its uniqueness.

- Notice that when you are focused on your stone, with appreciation, there is little room for regret or worry, for the past or the future. You are "at home" in the present moment.

REFLECTION

What did you notice when you anchored your awareness in your here-and-now stone?

When you were engaged with your stone, did your default mode activity—the wandering mind—lessen somewhat? If so, you can think of this as your "magic stone" because it can turn off your default mode network.

Going forward, you may want to keep your stone in your pocket. Whenever you get swept up in emotion, just rub your stone with your fingers. Feel the sensation of touching your stone. Enjoy it. Come home to the present moment.

INFORMAL PRACTICE

Mindfulness in Daily Life

- Mindfulness can be practiced every moment of the day—while you brush your teeth, while you walk from the parking garage to work, when you eat your breakfast, or whenever your cell phone rings.

  - *Pick an ordinary activity.* You might choose drinking your cup of coffee in the morning, taking a shower, or putting on your clothes. If you wish, select an activity that occurs early in the day before your attention is pulled in many directions.

  - *Choose one sensory experience* to explore in the activity, such as the sensation of taste as you drink your coffee or the sensation of water touching your body while showering.

- *Immerse yourself in the experience,* savoring it to the fullest. Return your mind to the sensations again and again when you notice it has wandered away.

- *Bring gentle, friendly awareness* to the activity until it has been completed.

• Try to bring mindful awareness to this activity every day for a week.

REFLECTION

Do you notice any way that bringing mindfulness into your everyday life changes things for you?

If you find it hard to practice meditation regularly, practicing a few minutes of mindfulness informally each day can also build the habit of being aware in the present moment. It's not a lesser practice, because in fact our goal is to bring awareness to as many moments of our lives as possible.

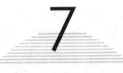

7

Letting Go of Resistance

Mindfulness doesn't just involve paying attention to what's happening in the present moment. It also involves a certain *quality* of attention—*accepting* what's happening, without being lost in judgments of good or bad. This attitude is often described as *nonresistance*. Resistance refers to the struggle that occurs when we believe our moment-to-moment experience should be other than it is.

For example, resistance to rush-hour traffic might look like this: *Damn it! The freeway is in total gridlock. I'm going to be late for dinner again! And I can't believe that stupid jerk just tried to cut in front of me from the on-ramp. I'm so sick of this I want to scream!!!*

Acceptance means that even though we may not *like* what's happening, we acknowledge that it *is* happening and can let go of the fact that things aren't exactly the way we want them to be.

Acceptance might look more like this: *Stuck in traffic yet again. Well, given that it's almost rush hour I guess that's to be expected. I'm certainly not going to get home any faster by being upset about it.*

How do we *know* when we're resisting? Some signs are being distracted, physically tense, getting lost in worry or rumination, overworking or overeating, feeling angry or irritated, or numbing out. These are ways we try to resist unwanted experiences. Resistance isn't all bad. Without resistance we would be overwhelmed by the intensity of our lives. Resistance can help us to function in the short term, but it can also have negative long-term consequences.

What we resist persists.

Unfortunately, when we resist unpleasant experiences, they don't typically go away; instead they just get worse. Have you ever had trouble getting to sleep at night when you know you have to be well rested for a big meeting the next day? What happens? Does fighting sleeplessness usually send you immediately off into peaceful slumber? Probably not. When we fight our difficult feelings, we just add fuel to their fire. *Resistance is futile* (as the aliens wisely tried to warn us).

> *Rafaella constantly struggled with anxiety, and she hated herself because of it. Whenever she felt anxious, she would try to force herself through the experience, telling herself, "Don't be such a baby. Grow up!" After a while, though, no matter how hard she fought, her body would become overwhelmed with anxiety, and she started to develop full-blown panic attacks.*

The meditation teacher Shinzen Young has a formula for this phenomenon:

$$\text{Suffering} = \text{Pain} \times \text{Resistance.}$$

In other words, pain in life—loss, worry, heartbreak, hardship—is inevitable, but when we resist the pain, it usually just makes the pain more intense. It's this add-on pain that can be equated with suffering. We suffer not only because it's painful in the moment, but because we bang our head against the wall of reality—getting frustrated because we think things should be other than they are.

Another common form of resistance is *denial*. We hope that if we don't think about a problem, it will go away. Research shows that when we try to suppress our unwanted thoughts or feelings, however, they just get stronger. Moreover, when we avoid or suppress painful thoughts and emotions, we can't see them clearly and respond with compassion.

What we can feel we can heal.

Mindfulness and self-compassion are resources that give us the safety needed to meet difficult experience with less resistance. Just imagine how you would feel if you were overwhelmed and a friend walked into the room, gave you a hug, sat down beside you, listened to your distress, and then helped you work out a plan of action. Thankfully, that mindful and compassionate friend can be you. It begins by opening to what is, without resistance.

Given that mindfulness is a core component of self-compassion, it's worth asking the question "How do mindfulness and self-compassion relate to one another?" Are they the same or different?

From our point of view, although the two are closely intertwined, there are some differences:

- Mindfulness focuses primarily on acceptance of *experience*. Self-compassion focuses more on caring for the *experiencer*.

- Mindfulness asks, "What am I *experiencing* right now?" Self-compassion asks, "What do I *need* right now?"

- Mindfulness says, "*Feel* your suffering with spacious awareness." Self-compassion says, "*Be kind to yourself* when you suffer."

Despite the differences, both mindfulness and self-compassion allow us to live with *less resistance* toward ourselves and our lives. The central paradox of mindful self-compassion training can be summed up like this:

When we struggle, we give ourselves compassion not to feel better but *because* we feel bad.

In other words, we can't just throw self-compassion at ourselves as a way to make the pain go away. If we do, we're engaging in a hidden form of resistance that will ultimately just make things worse. However, if we can fully accept that things *are* painful, and be kind to ourselves *because* they're painful, we can be with the pain with greater ease. We need mindfulness to ensure that self-compassion isn't used in the service of resistance, and we need self-compassion to feel safe and secure enough to mindfully open to difficult experiences. Together they form a beautiful dance.

After practicing speaking to herself compassionately for some months, Rafaella learned to hold herself and her anxiety with mindfulness and compassion, rather than fighting the experience. When Rafaella became anxious or even a little panicky, her inner dialogue went something like this, spoken from a compassionate part of herself: "I know you feel really scared right now. I wish things weren't so difficult, but they are. I know there is tightening in your throat and some dizziness in your head. Still, I care for you and I'm here for you. You are not alone. We'll get through this." With a new, more compassionate inner voice, Rafaella's panic attacks receded and she found she was much more capable of working with her anxiety than she had realized.

 EXERCISE
The Ice Cube

This exercise is an opportunity to experience resistance in real time, as well as what might happen when we apply mindfulness and compassion to the experience of resistance. Read through the instructions and decide whether this is a good time for you to try it.

- The exercise should be conducted outside or on a waterproof floor. (People with Raynaud's disease are advised against doing this exercise.)

- Get one or two ice cubes from the freezer and hold them in your closed hand as long as possible. Keep holding them.

- After a few minutes, notice what thoughts come into your mind (e.g., this will harm me, I can't bear this, the people who created this exercise are cruel!). That's *resistance*.

- Now pay close attention to what you are experiencing, moment to moment. For example, feel the *sensation* of cold as simply cold. If pain sensations are pulsing up your arm, feel the pulsations as pulsations. Notice your *emotions,* such as fear, as simply fear. Notice any impulse to action that may be arising, such as to drop the ice and open your palm to alleviate the cold. Let yourself be aware of your impulses as simply impulses. That's *mindfulness*.

- Now let's add a little *kindness* to the mix. For example, let yourself be comforted by the thought that this exercise hurts, but it isn't harmful. You can let out a long exhalation of relief . . . *ahhhhh*. If you notice any discomfort in your hand, maybe add a sound of tenderness . . . *awwww*. Appreciate your hand for alerting you to the sensation of pain. Also, give yourself a nod of respect or admiration for enduring this exercise to learn something new. It took courage.

- You can finally release the ice cube!

REFLECTION

What did you notice while doing this practice? What came up for you? Did mindfulness or self-kindness change your experience in any way?

For many people, this exercise offers a powerful taste of how resistance can amplify pain. It also illustrates how when we mindfully accept our pain and offer ourselves kindness because it hurts, our suffering may diminish. If you weren't able to let go of your natural resistance to the cold of the ice cube, however, don't blame yourself. Your resistance stems from your natural desire to be safe. But also within you lies the ability to feel safe through your own care, support, and comfort. You just may need to be a bit patient as you work to temper your automatic reactions.

 EXERCISE
How Do I Cause Myself Unnecessary Suffering?

- Think of a current situation in your life where you feel that resisting the reality of something painful is causing you unnecessary suffering and may actually be making things worse than they need to be (e.g., procrastinating on a big project, resenting something about your current job, harboring anger toward your neighbor's barking dog). Then write it down.

- *How do you know that you are resisting?* Is there any discomfort in the body or the mind? Can you describe it?

- *What are the consequences of resisting?* For example, how might your life be easier if you stopped resisting or at least resisted a little less?

- *Can you see that resistance might be serving you in some way?* Perhaps resistance is helping you not to feel certain feelings that could be overwhelming. If difficult feelings arise, be kind to yourself. Honor your resistance, knowing that sometimes it allows you to function in the world.

- *Now consider how mindfulness or self-compassion might help lessen your resistance in this situation.* Might validating the pain ("This is tough") and letting it into your life ("opening the hand of fear") make things easier or more difficult? Or would offering yourself a little understanding ("It's not your fault") or remembering common humanity ("This is how people feel in these situations") bring some relief?

REFLECTION

Some people feel a bit vulnerable after doing this exercise. Letting go of our resistance means opening to pain, and it's hard to open to pain. It may require acknowledging that we often don't have as much control over the events of our lives as we would like. This is where we need to give ourselves great kindness and compassion. If you're feeling at all upset after doing this exercise, try putting a hand over your heart or some other soothing place and saying some supportive words to yourself. What would you say to a friend who was feeling like you are at the moment? Can you try saying something similar to yourself?

 INFORMAL PRACTICE
Noticing Resistance

Because resisting pain is so natural and automatic (even an amoeba will move away from a toxin in a petri dish), most of our resistance goes unnoticed. A very useful practice, for this reason, is simply noticing when we're resisting and labeling it when it happens.

For the next week, see if you can notice any small moments when you are resisting something unpleasant (you don't want to go to your Tuesday night aerobics class, the elevator at work is broken and you have to take the stairs yet again, your teenage son left his dirty dishes on the counter for you to wash, and so on). When you notice resistance is occurring, simply use a neutral, matter-of-fact tone of voice to label it: "Resistance." "This is a moment of resistance."

The more we can notice when we're resisting, the less unnecessary tension and stress we will allow into our lives and the better our chances of behaving wisely in difficult situations.

8

Backdraft

Backdraft refers to the pain—often very old pain—that may arise when we give ourselves kindness and compassion. The experience of backdraft can be confusing for some people, but it is a key part of the transformation process—growing pains.

Backdraft is a term that firefighters use to describe what happens when a fire has used all available oxygen and fresh oxygen is introduced through an open window or door. The air rushes in and the flames rush out. A similar effect can occur when we open the door of our hearts with self-compassion. Most of our hearts are hot with suffering accumulated over a lifetime. To function in our lives, we have needed to shut out stressful or painful experiences to protect ourselves. This means that when we open the door of our hearts and the fresh air of self-compassion flows in, old pain and fear is likely to come out. That's backdraft.

> *Chad was encouraged by his first two self-compassion classes, but then he started doubting whether he was doing it right. Whenever he put his hands on his heart and tried to speak kindly to himself, he felt queasy and anxious and short of breath. "What's wrong with me?" Chad wondered. "Shouldn't this make me feel* better?*"*

It's important to realize that the discomfort of backdraft is not *created* by self-compassion practice. We aren't doing anything wrong when we experience backdraft. In fact, it's a sign that we're doing it right, we're starting to open the door of our hearts. At first, however, we may reexperience old pain as it starts to be released. This is a natural process and nothing to be worried about.

> *Backdraft is a sign that the healing process has begun.*

How Do We Recognize Backdraft?

Backdraft can show up as any type of emotional, mental, or physical uneasiness.
For example:

- *Emotionally*—shame, grief, fear, sadness

- *Mentally*—thoughts like "I'm all alone," "I'm a failure," "I'm unworthy"

- *Physically*—body memories, aches, pains

Often uneasiness appears out of nowhere, and we may not understand why
it's happening. Tears can appear while meditating, or anger, or a sense of fear and
vulnerability. And a whole chain of reactions can be set off when we struggle not
to feel backdraft. For example, we might go into our heads (intellectualize), become
agitated, withdraw, space out, or criticize ourselves and others. All these reactions
can (and should) be met with kindness and compassion. The important thing is that
we don't let ourselves become overwhelmed with feelings of backdraft, but allow
ourselves to open the door of our heart slowly.

You need to be self-compassionate whenever backdraft arises, allowing yourself
to go at your own pace.

WHAT CAN WE DO ABOUT BACKDRAFT?

> *Ask yourself,*
> *"What do I need to*
> *feel safe right now?"*

You can begin by asking yourself, "What do I need right
now?"—especially "What do I need to feel *safe*?" Then,
depending on what feels right to you, you may consider
any of the following strategies:

Practice Mindfulness to Regulate Attention

◇ Label the experience as backdraft—"Oh, this is 'backdraft'"—in the tone you might
use with a dear friend.

◇ Name your strongest emotion and validate it for yourself in a compassionate manner ("Ah, that's *grief*").

◇ Explore where the emotion physically resides in your body, perhaps as tension in
your stomach or hollowness in your heart, and give that part of your body soothing
or supportive touch.

◇ Redirect your attention to a neutral focus inside your body (e.g., the breath) or a
sense object in the outside world (e.g., ambient sounds, your here-and-now stone—
see Chapter 6). The farther you direct your attention from your body, the easier it
will be.

◇ Feel the soles of your feet (see the next page).

Take Refuge in Ordinary Activities

- You may feel the need to anchor your awareness in some everyday activity, such as washing the dishes, going for a walk, showering, or doing exercise. If you happen to find the activity pleasant or rewarding for your senses (smell, taste, touch, sound, vision), allow yourself to savor it. (See "Mindfulness in Daily Life," Chapter 6.)

- Or you may feel the need to comfort, soothe, or support yourself in a practical, behavioral way, such as by having a cup of tea or a warm bath, listening to music, or petting your dog. (See "Self-Compassion in Daily Life" on the next page.)

- If you need further help, make use of your personal support system (friends, family, therapists, teachers) to get what you need.

Once Chad learned about backdraft, he wasn't so upset when it happened. When anxiety arose, he told himself, "Oh, that's backdraft; that's normal." He even knew the source of his backdraft. His mother drank a bit too much while he was growing up, and although she was usually loving and nurturing, she would occasionally snap at him and get angry for no reason. He learned as a child that he couldn't completely count on her love and support—it partly depended on how much wine she had had. He realized that when he gave himself love and support, old feelings of insecurity would arise. Sometimes just labeling it was enough to keep him from becoming anxious and short of breath. At other times the backdraft was stronger, and Chad knew the kindest thing to do was to pull back. "Let me try just feeling the soles of my feet. That helps to make me feel grounded." Occasionally Chad felt overwhelmed by more intense emotions—fear and disgust—and he knew to just stop the practice for a while and do something ordinary and pleasant, like taking a bicycle ride along the beach. Later, when Chad felt better, he returned to intentional self-compassion practices like putting his hand on his heart in a curious, exploratory way, not expecting to feel any particular way.

INFORMAL PRACTICE
Feeling the Soles of Your Feet

This practice is designed to stabilize and ground you when you are experiencing overwhelming emotions or backdraft. Research shows this practice can help regulate strong emotions such as anger.

- Stand up and feel the soles of your feet on the floor. This can be done with or without shoes.

- Begin to notice the sensations—the sense of touch—in the soles of your feet on the floor.

- To better feel sensation in the soles of the feet, try gently rocking forward and backward on your feet, and side to side. Try making little circles with your knees, feeling the changing sensations in the soles of your feet.

- When the mind has wandered, just feel the soles of your feet again.

- Now begin to walk, slowly, noticing the changing sensations in the soles of your feel. Notice the sensation of lifting a foot, stepping forward, and then placing the foot on the floor. Now do the same with the other foot. And then one foot after another.

- As you walk, appreciate how small the surface area of each foot is and how your feet support your entire body. If you wish, allow a moment of gratitude for the hard work that your feet are doing, which we usually take for granted.

- Continue to walk, slowly, feeling the soles of your feet.

- Now return to standing again and expand your awareness to your entire body, letting yourself feel whatever you're feeling and letting yourself be just as you are.

REFLECTION

What did you notice while doing this practice? What came up for you?

There are many reasons this practice is so effective when you're feeling emotionally overwhelmed. First of all, your attention is focused on the soles of your feet—as far away as possible from your head (where the story line of what's happening resides). Also, feeling that point of contact with the earth can help you feel supported and grounded, literally. You might like to take your shoes off and do this practice on the grass, when possible, so the connection with the earth can be felt even more palpably. Feel free to practice "soles of the feet" wherever you happen to be when difficult emotions arise—in line at the airport security checkpoint, walking down the hall at work, and so on.

 INFORMAL PRACTICE
Self-Compassion in Daily Life

- It's important to remember that you already know how to be self-compassionate. You would not have lived this long if you couldn't care for yourself. Self-*care* in the midst of difficulty is self-*compassion*—a kindly response to suffering. Therefore, anyone can learn self-compassion.

- Self-compassion is much more than training the mind. *Behavioral* self-compassion is a safe and effective way of practicing self-compassion. It anchors self-compassion practice in ordinary activities of daily life.

- If you find that you are experiencing a lot of backdraft when practicing self-compassion in explicit ways (such as giving yourself soothing touch), you can find more ordinary ways to practice self-compassion that feel safer.

- Fill out this list of ways you already care for yourself, thinking of some new possibilities you might add to your repertoire.

- Try doing any of these activities as a way of being kind to yourself in a moment of struggle.

Physically—Soften the Body

How do you care for yourself physically (e.g., exercise, massage, warm bath, cup of tea)?

Can you think of new ways to release the tension and stress that build up in your body?

Mentally—Reduce Agitation

How do you care for your mind, especially when you're under stress (e.g., meditate, watch a funny movie, read an inspiring book)?

Is there a new strategy you'd like to try to let your thoughts come and go more easily?

Emotionally—Soothe and Comfort Yourself

How do you care for yourself emotionally (pet the dog, journal, cook)?

Is there something new you'd like to try?

Relationally—Connect with Others

How or when do you relate to others in ways that bring you genuine happiness (e.g., meet with friends, send a birthday card, play a game)?

Is there any way that you'd like to enrich these connections?

Spiritually—Commit to Your Values

What do you do to care for yourself spiritually (pray, walk in the woods, help others)?

Is there anything else you'd like to remember to do to help nurture your spiritual side?

9

Developing Loving-Kindness

In addition to learning how to deepen our self-compassion practice, it is important to develop feelings of loving-kindness toward ourselves more generally. *Loving-kindness* is the English translation of the Pali term *metta,* which is also translated as "friendliness."

How are compassion and loving-kindness different? Compassion may be defined as "sensitivity to the pain or suffering of another, coupled with a deep desire to alleviate that suffering." Self-compassion is simply compassion directed toward one-self—*inner* compassion. Loving-kindness entails general feelings of friendliness to oneself and others and doesn't necessarily involve suffering. It's important that we cultivate a generally friendly stance toward ourselves, even when things are going well in the moment.

According to the Dalai Lama, loving-kindness is "the wish that all sentient beings may be *happy.*" Compassion is "the wish that all sentient beings may be *free from suffering.*" A meditation teacher from Myanmar put it this way: "When the sunshine of loving-kindness meets the tears of suffering, the rainbow of compassion arises."

> *When loving-kindness bumps into suffering and stays loving, it becomes compassion. Both are expressions of* goodwill.

Metta can be developed in a practice called *loving-kindness meditation.* In this practice the meditator thinks of a particular person, visualizes her, and silently repeats a series of phrases designed to evoke feelings of goodwill toward that person. Examples of common phrases are "May you be happy," "May you be peaceful," "May you be healthy," "May you live with ease." The phrases can be thought of as friendly wishes or good intentions.

Typically, meditators start by directing the phrases to themselves, then aim the phrases of goodwill toward a mentor or benefactor, then someone they feel neutral about, then someone toward whom they have difficult feelings, and finally the idea is to expand the circle of loving-kindness to include all sentient beings. The good intentions cultivated by loving-kindness meditation lead to more supportive self-talk and better moods. Research shows that loving-kindness meditation is "dose dependent"—the more you do, the more powerful the effects. One of the key benefits of loving-kindness meditation is reduced negative emotions like anxiety and depression and increased positive emotions like happiness and joy.

Some people struggle with loving-kindness meditation because they find the process of repeating phrases clumsy or awkward, or they discontinue the practice because the phrases sound robotic or inauthentic. If you have this experience, don't worry. There is a story from the Judaic tradition that illustrates how the practice works:

> A disciple asks the rabbi, "Why does Torah tell us to 'place these words upon your hearts'? Why does it not tell us to place these holy words in our hearts?"
>
> The rabbi answers, "It is because as we are, our hearts are closed, and we cannot place the holy words in our hearts. So we place them on top of our hearts. And there they stay until, one day, the heart breaks and the words fall in."

 MEDITATION
Loving-Kindness for a Loved One

Traditionally, loving-kindness meditation starts with kindness toward oneself. "Love your neighbor as (you love) yourself." In modern times we reverse the order, beginning with someone else whom we naturally love, and then we sneak ourselves in. Many people use this variant of loving-kindness meditation as their primary meditation practice. (A guided recording of this meditation can be found online; see the end of the Contents for information.)

- Allow yourself to settle into a comfortable position, either sitting or lying down. If you like, put a hand over your heart or another location that is soothing as a reminder to bring not only awareness, but loving awareness to your experience and to yourself.

A Living Being That Makes You Smile

- Bring to mind a person or other living being who naturally makes you smile—someone with whom you have an easy, uncomplicated relationship. This could be a child, your grandmother, your cat or dog—whoever naturally brings happiness to your heart. If many people or other living beings arise, just choose one.

- Let yourself feel what it's like to be in that being's presence. Allow yourself to enjoy the good company. Create a vivid image of this being in your mind's eye.

May You . . .

- Now, recognize how this being wishes to be happy and free from suffering, just like you and every other living being. Repeat silently, feeling the importance of your words:
  - *May you be happy.*
  - *May you be peaceful.*
  - *May you be healthy.*
  - *May you live with ease.*

(Repeat several times, slowly and gently.)

- You may wish to use your own phrases if you have ones you normally work with, or continue to repeat these phrases.

- When you notice that your mind has wandered, return to the words and the image of the loved one you have in mind. Savor any warm feelings that may arise. Take your time.

May You and I (We) . . .

- Now add *yourself* to your circle of goodwill. Create an image of yourself in the presence of your loved one, visualizing you both together.
  - *May you and I be happy.*
  - *May you and I be peaceful.*
  - *May you and I be healthy.*
  - *May you and I live with ease.*

(Repeat several times, using "we" rather than "you and I" if you like.)

- Now let go of the image of the other, perhaps thanking your loved one before moving on, and then letting the full focus of your attention rest directly on yourself.

May I . . .

- Put your hand over your heart, or elsewhere, and feel the warmth and gentle pressure of your hand. Visualize your whole body in your mind's eye, noticing any stress or uneasiness that may be lingering within you, and offering yourself the phrases.
  - *May I be happy.*
  - *May I be peaceful.*

- *May I be healthy.*

- *May I live with ease.*

(Repeat several times, with warmth.)

• Finally, take a few breaths and just rest quietly in your own body, accepting whatever your experience is, exactly as it is.

REFLECTION

What did you notice during this meditation? What came up for you? Was it easier to feel loving-kindness toward your loved one than yourself? How was it to direct the feelings of loving-kindness to both of you together? Were there any challenging aspects to this meditation? Could you hold that in compassion?

It's common for people to find that it's a lot easier to feel loving-kindness for a loved one than for themselves. In this meditation, we start with an easy person to activate the energy of loving-kindness, and then we "tuck ourselves in" to keep the flow of loving-kindness going toward a more difficult person—ourselves.

Many people still struggle with loving-kindness meditation, however. The phrases just don't ring true, or perhaps words like "May I" sound strange or feel awkward. In the next chapter, we will help you find your own loving-kindness phrases that feel more meaningful and authentic.

 INFORMAL PRACTICE
Walking in Loving-Kindness

We can practice the attitude of loving-kindness throughout the day by directing phrases of goodwill toward ourselves or anyone we meet. *Note:* This informal practice uses the act of walking to ground our awareness, but people who move using a wheelchair or other device may use any point of bodily contact as a substitute for the sensation of walking.

- Whenever you are outdoors walking down the street, or in a busy place like a shopping center, you can try this practice.

- First, pay attention to your own feet as you walk, noticing the sensations in your feet and legs (no need to walk at a slow pace).

- As you walk, begin silently repeating the phrase, "May *I* be happy and free from suffering."

- Then, when you notice or pass by another person, silently offer them a kind phrase, such as "May *you* be happy and free from suffering," seeing if you can also connect to some warmth or goodwill toward that person.

- If it feels safe and appropriate, you might try giving a nod or a light smile to the people you meet, silently repeating, "May *you* be happy and free from suffering."

- Whenever you feel distracted or uncomfortable, just redirect your attention to the sensations in your feet and legs and say to yourself, "May *I* be happy and free from suffering." And when the time is right, return your attention to others.

- Finally, see if you can expand your friendly wishes to include everyone within your field of vision—all living things—and don't forget yourself! Repeat silently, "May *all beings* be happy and free from suffering."

REFLECTION

What did you notice while doing this practice? Did your perceptions of other people change? Did their reactions to you change?

This practice can be a powerful way of generating a sense of connection with all beings. It can be used in a store or restaurant, while commuting to work in a car or train—any place we go where there are other people.

If the phrase "May I/you be happy and free from suffering" doesn't evoke genuine feelings of kindness and compassion within you, wait to do this practice until you discover your own authentic phrases in the next chapter.

10

Loving-Kindness for Ourselves

To experience the benefits of loving-kindness meditation, sometimes it's necessary to personalize the practice. The purpose of this chapter, therefore, is to help you find loving-kindness phrases that really speak to you, a unique key that can unlock the door of your own heart.

Ushi was a dedicated meditation practitioner and had been doing loving-kindness practice for years—ever since she learned it from one of her favorite teachers on a retreat. She had a dirty little secret, however. Whenever she said her loving-kindness phrases she felt nothing, like a robot repeating words mechanically with no feeling whatsoever. She suspected that maybe she just didn't have the right temperament to feel loving-kindness.

> *The benefits of loving-kindness meditation come to us when we personalize the practice.*

Many of the traditional loving-kindness phrases used in meditation have been handed down over centuries, so it's not surprising they can be a bit hard to connect with. For this reason, it is important to find loving-kindness phrases that resonate. This is especially true when we want to generate feelings of loving-kindness for ourselves—they must feel authentic to have impact.

Finding phrases is like writing poetry, which may be described as finding words to express something that cannot be put into words. Our aim is to find language that evokes the energy or attitude of loving-kindness and compassion.

Just as the breath can be an anchor for meditation, loving-kindness phrases can also anchor our awareness. The calming aspect of meditation comes from concentration, so if you can settle on two to four phrases that you would like to repeat over and over, that will support the concentrative aspect of meditation. Loving-kindness phrases can also be used during everyday life, however, as we saw in the Walking in

Loving-Kindness practice (see Chapter 9). You can be more flexible with the phrases you use in daily life, changing things up according to what feels right in the moment.

There are a few guidelines for finding loving-kindness phrases that are deeply meaningful to you:

- The phrases should be *simple, clear, authentic,* and *kind.* There should be no argument in the mind when we offer ourselves a loving-kindness phrase, only gratitude: "Oh, thank you! Thank you."

- You don't need to use "may I" phrases if they feel awkward, or too much like begging. Loving-kindness phrases are *wishes.* "May I" is simply an invitation to *incline the heart* in a positive direction. It means "That it would be so" or "If all the conditions would allow it to be so, then. . . ." Loving-kindness phrases are like blessings.

- The phrases *are not positive affirmations* (e.g., "I'm becoming healthier every day"). We are simply cultivating good intentions, not pretending things are other than they are.

- The phrases are designed to evoke *goodwill, not good feelings.* A common reason for difficulty with loving-kindness meditation is that we have expectations about how we're supposed to feel. Loving-kindness practice doesn't directly change our emotions. However, good *feelings* are an inevitable byproduct of *goodwill.*

- *The phrases should be general.* For example, "May I be healthy" rather than "May I be free from my diabetes."

- The phrases should be *said slowly*: there's no rush—the most phrases said in the shortest time doesn't win the race!

- The phrases should be said warmly, like whispering them into the ear of someone you truly love. What matters most is the *attitude* behind the phrases.

- Finally, you may address yourself as "I," "you," or using your proper name ("George"). You may also use a term of endearment, such as "Sweetheart" or "Dear One." Addressing yourself in this way supports the attitude of kindness and compassion.

> *Loving-kindness phrases should focus on the question "What do I need?"*

What Do I Need?

One way to find authentic and meaningful phrases is to focus on the core question of self-compassion training: "What do I *need*?"

What is a *need*, and what is the difference between needs and wants? *Wants* are personal and arise from the neck up—in the head. They are infinite, such as wanting a special brand of coffee or a fancy car. *Needs* are more universal and arise (metaphorically) from the neck down. Examples of human needs are the need to be accepted, validated, seen, heard, protected, loved, known, cherished, connected, or respected. There are other needs that are still universal but perhaps less relational, such as the need for health, growth, freedom, humor, integrity, or safety. Discovering what we truly need is the basis for finding genuinely meaningful loving-kindness phrases for ourselves.

When Ushi finally created her own loving-kindness phrases—sending wishes to herself that spoke to her deepest needs—it was transformative. The three phrases she settled on were "May I be courageous. May I be seen for who I truly am. May I live in love." Instead of simply repeating the words robotically, each phrase resonated with meaning for her. Now, most every time Ushi practices loving-kindness meditation, she feels as if she is giving herself a precious gift and receiving it with an open, grateful heart.

EXERCISE
Finding Loving-Kindness Phrases

This exercise is designed to help you discover loving-kindness and compassion phrases that are deeply meaningful to you. If you already have phrases and wish to continue using them, try this exercise as an experiment and don't feel you need to change your phrases. (An audio guide to this exercise is available online; see the end of the Contents for information.)

What Do I Need?

- To start, please put a hand over your heart, or elsewhere, and feel your body breathe.

- Now take a moment and allow your heart to open gently—to become receptive—like a flower opens in the warm sun.

- Then ask yourself this question, allowing the answer to arise naturally within you:

  - "What do I need?" "What do I *truly* need?"

  - If this need has not been fulfilled in a given day, your day does not feel complete.

  - Let the answer be a *universal* human need, such as the need to be connected, loved, peaceful, free.

- When you are ready, write down what arose for you.

- The words you discovered can be used in meditation just as they are, like a mantra, or you can rewrite them as wishes for yourself, such as:

- *May I be kind to myself*
- *May I begin to be kind to myself*
- *May I know that I belong*
- *May I live in peace*
- *May I rest in love*

What Do I Need to *Hear*?

- Now consider a second question:
  - *What do I need to hear from others?* What words do I long to hear because, as a person, *I really need to hear words like this?* Open the door of your heart and wait for words to come.
  - If I could, *what words would I like to have whispered into my ear* every day for the rest of my life—words that might make me say, "Oh, thank you, thank you" every time I hear them? Allow yourself to be vulnerable and open to this possibility, with courage. Listen.
- Now, when you're ready, write down what you heard.

- If you heard a *lot* of words, see if you can make the words into a short phrase—*a message to yourself.*

- The words you wrote down can also be used in loving-kindness meditation just as they are, or you can also rewrite them as *wishes for yourself.* Actually, words that we would like to hear from others again and again are *qualities we would like to actualize* in our own lives. For example, longing to hear "I love you" probably means that we wish to know we are truly lovable. That's why we need to hear the words over and over again.

What Do You Want to Know for Sure?

- If you like, you can reframe your words as wishes for yourself. For example:
  - "I love you" can become the wish "May I love myself just as I am."
  - "I'm here for you" can become the wish "May I feel safe and secure."
  - "You're a good person" can become the wish "May I know my own goodness."

- Now, take a moment to review what you have written and settle on two to four words or phrases you would like to use in meditation, then write them down. These words or phrases are gifts you will give to yourself over and over again.

- Take a moment to *memorize* these words or phrases.

- Finally, try them out to see how they land. Begin saying your phrases over and over, slowly and gently, *whispering* them into your own ear as if into the ear of a loved one. Perhaps *hearing* the words from the inside, allowing them to resonate within you. Allowing the words to *take up space,* to *fill your being.*

- Then gently *release* the phrases and allow yourself to rest in the experience, letting this practice be just what it was and letting yourself be just as you are.

- Consider this exercise to be only the beginning of a search for phrases that are just right for you. Finding loving-kindness phrases is a soulful journey, a poetic journey. Hopefully you will find yourself returning to this process ("What do I need? What do I long to hear?") as you practice loving-kindness meditation.

REFLECTION

What did you notice while you did this exercise? Were you surprised by what you needed? How do you feel about the phrases that emerged?

How do we know when we have found a good phrase? Gratitude! With gratitude there is no more longing. We are complete. The heart is at rest. It may take a while to find phrases that work for you like that, but it's worth the effort.

MEDITATION
Loving-Kindness for Ourselves

In this meditation, you will use the phrases you discovered in the Finding Loving-Kindness Phrases exercise. Review your phrases and decide which ones you will use rather than taking the meditation time to find new phrases. (A guided recording of this meditation is available online; see the end of the Contents for information.)

Loving-kindness meditation has many elements, and practitioners generally try too hard to get it right. To counter this tendency, see if you can give up the wish to feel anything in particular during the meditation. Just allow the words to do all the work, much like slipping into a warm bath and letting the water do its magic.

- Find a comfortable position, sitting or lying down. Let your eyes close, fully or partially. Take a few deep breaths to settle into your body and into the present moment.

- Put your hand over your heart, or wherever it is comforting and soothing, as a reminder to bring not only awareness, but *loving* awareness, to your experience and to yourself.

- After a while, feel your breath move in your body, wherever you notice it most easily. Feel the gentle rhythm of your breathing, and when your attention wanders, notice the gentle movement of your breath once again.

- Now, release the focus on your breath, allow the breath to slip into the background of your awareness, and begin to offer yourself the phrases that are most meaningful to you.

- Repeat the words over and over, letting them encircle you—surrounding yourself with words of love and compassion.

- If it feels right, absorb the words, letting them fill your being. Allow the words to resonate in every cell of your body.

- Nothing to do, nowhere to go. Just bathe yourself with kind words, soaking them up—words that you need to hear.

- And whenever you notice that your mind has wandered, you can refresh your aim by offering yourself soothing touch, or just by feeling the sensations in your body. And then offer yourself the words. Come home to kindness.

- Finally, release the phrases and rest quietly in your own body.

REFLECTION

What did you notice while doing this meditation? Did you feel more connected to the practice by using personalized phrases? How are you feeling now?

Many people find that they are able to feel the meaning of their phrases more easily once they have found the right words. If the practice still feels awkward, however, you might try reducing the number of words you are using. Perhaps just using a few single words, like "love," "support," "acceptance," and the like, will feel more natural. Play with it until you find something that works for you.

This is the second core meditation of the MSC course, so try it out for about 20 minutes for a few days in a row to see if you get the hang of it. As mentioned before, we recommend you do some combination of formal (meditation) and informal (daily life) practice for about 30 minutes per day.

And if it seems like loving-kindness meditation never quite resonates, that's okay too. There are many different practices and meditations in the workbook to help you cultivate a compassionate relationship with yourself. The main thing is that you set your intention to bring more kindness into your life in a manner that feels just right for you.

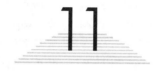

Self-Compassionate Motivation

One of the biggest blocks to self-compassion is the belief that it will undermine our motivation. We fear that if we're kind to ourselves, we won't have the drive needed to make changes or reach our goals. The thinking is "If I'm too self-compassionate, won't I just sit around all day surfing the Internet and eating junk food?" Well, does a compassionate mother who cares about her teenage son let him do whatever he wants (like sit around all day surfing the Internet and eating junk food)? Of course not. She tells him to go to school, do his homework, and get to bed on time. Why would it be any different for *self*-compassion?

And what if the mother wants to *motivate* her child to make necessary changes? Let's say her teenage son comes home from school with a failing math grade. She has choices for how to help him improve. One way is with harsh criticism: "I'm ashamed of you. You're a loser. You'll never amount to anything." Makes you cringe, doesn't it? (Yet don't we say some pretty awful things to ourselves when we fail or feel inadequate?) And does it work? Temporarily perhaps. The boy might work harder for a while to escape his mother's wrath, but in the long term he'll no doubt lose confidence in his ability to do math and become afraid of failure, and he won't sign up for advanced math courses any time soon.

> *Self-compassion does not make us lazy.*

Bill was a highly successful computer engineer in Silicon Valley. Top of his class at UC Berkeley, he was now thinking of launching his own business where he could create software that was exciting and innovative. The way Bill had always motivated himself to succeed was with relentless self-criticism. When he received an A– on an exam in college, for instance, he would cut himself down mercilessly. "What kind of loser are you? If you aren't at the top of your class, you're a failure. You should be ashamed that you didn't get an A." He still used this approach to motivate himself as an adult, and he truly believed that if he were not harsh with himself, he would turn into a slacker.

Lately, Bill had begun having intense anxiety whenever he tried to move forward with his new business. What if he didn't succeed? What if this new project proved to everyone that he was a failure? An imposter? A fake? Bill got himself so worked up about the price of failure and his life became so unhappy that the only relief came when he considered giving up on his dream.

But there is another way the mother can motivate her son, help him bounce back from failure and succeed—by giving him compassion. For example, "Oh, dear, you must be so upset. Come here, let me give you a hug. You know I love you no matter what." That tells her son that he's acceptable even when he fails. But a compassionate mother doesn't stop there if she truly cares about her son's well-being. There's an action component. She's likely to add something like "I know you want to go to college and, of course, you need to do well on your entrance exams to get in. What can I do to help you? I know you can do it if you work hard enough. I believe in you."

This type of encouragement and support is likely to be much more effective and sustainable in the long run. Research shows that self-compassionate people not only have greater self-confidence, but they are less likely to fear failure and are more likely to try again when they do fail, and to persist in their efforts to keep learning.

> *The motivation of self-compassion arises from love, while the motivation of self-criticism arises from fear. Love is more powerful than fear.*

Still, it's important to understand *why* we criticize ourselves. It hurts like hell, so why do we do it?

As mentioned in Chapter 4, self-criticism is rooted in the threat-defense system. At some level, our inner critic is trying to force us to change so that we'll be *safe*. For example, why would we beat ourselves up for being out of shape? Because we're afraid our bodies are going to fall apart and stop working properly. Why do we criticize ourselves for procrastinating on an important task at work? So we can avoid failing, losing our job, and becoming homeless. At some level, our inner critic is constantly trying to ward off dangers that might cause us harm. Of course, the inner critic may not be helpful at all—this approach may be completely counterproductive—but its intentions are often good. With this understanding, we can start to transform the critical voice within us so it's not so harsh and unforgiving. We can learn to motivate ourselves with a *new* voice—that of the *compassionate self.*

It was initially quite difficult for Bill to become more self-compassionate because of his fear that going easier on himself would make him work less and abandon his goals. Ironically, the reality was quite the opposite. Bill's inner critic was so harsh that he dreaded the possibility of failure and he couldn't see his way around simple challenges. So he started to seriously procrastinate about taking even small steps toward his dream. Bill knew his merciless inner voice was part of the problem, and he decided that something had to change if he was to make any progress.

At the time, Bill had a trainer at the gym who was about his age and who was endlessly supportive. For example, when Bill collapsed while doing push-ups, his trainer just said, "Great! Working to the point of muscle exhaustion is what we want," and when Bill wanted to lift weights that might have injured him, his coach said, "Hey Bill, let's save that one for later. We'll get there sooner than you think." So Bill decided to apply the same attitude to his new business project. "Just give it a try," he told himself. "I know you can do it." And he imagined what his trainer would say when a setback occurred: "Hang in there, bro. We've got this." Bill slowly began to discover his compassionate voice and learned how to support rather than sabotage himself. Eventually he quit his company job, found the venture capital needed to start his new project, and started living the life he needed to live—one that made him happy.

EXERCISE
Finding Your Compassionate Voice

This exercise will help you hear the critical voice inside, discover how your inner critic may be trying to help you, and learn to motivate yourself with a new voice—that of your inner compassionate self.

Sometimes the inner critic does not appear to have our best interests in mind. This can especially be true if our inner critic is the internalized voice of someone from our past who was abusive. Please be compassionate with yourself as you do this exercise. If you find yourself getting into uncomfortable territory, let it go and return to it only when you feel strong and ready. You might wish to reread the "Tips for Practice" in the Introduction before doing this exercise.

> *Ask yourself, "What do I need right now?"*

- In the space provided below and on the next page, write down a *behavior* that you would like to change—something you often beat yourself up about. Choose a behavior that is unhelpful to you and is causing you unhappiness, but for this exercise, select a behavior in the mild to moderate range of difficulty. Also, pick a behavior that is potentially changeable. (Don't choose a permanent characteristic like "My feet are too big.") Examples are "I'm impatient," "I don't exercise enough," "I procrastinate."

Identifying Your Self-Critical Voice

- Write down what you typically say to yourself when you engage in this behavior. Sometimes the inner critic is harsh, but sometimes it manifests more as a discouraged feeling or in some other way. What *words* does it use, and importantly, what *tone* does it use? Or perhaps there are no words at all, but an image. How does your inner critic express itself?

- Now, take a moment to notice how it *feels* when you criticize yourself. Consider how much distress the voice of self-criticism has caused you. If you wish, try giving yourself compassion for how hard it is to hear such harsh language, perhaps by validating the pain: "This is hard." "I'm so sorry, I know how much it hurts to hear this."

- Reflect for a moment on *why* the criticism has gone on for so long. Is your inner critic trying to protect you in some way, to keep you safe from danger, to help you, even if the result has been unproductive? If so, write down what you think might be motivating your inner critic.

- If you can't find any way that your critical voice is trying to help you— sometimes self-criticism has no redeeming value whatsoever—please don't go further and simply continue to give yourself compassion for how you've suffered from it in the past.

  If you did identify some way your inner critic might be trying to help you or keep you safe, however, see if you can acknowledge its efforts, perhaps even writing down a *few words of thanks*. Let your inner critic know that even though it may not be serving you very well now, its intention was good, and it was doing its best.

Finding Your Compassionate Voice

- Now that your self-critical voice has been heard, see if you can make some space for another voice—your inner *compassionate voice*. This comes from a part of yourself that is very wise and recognizes how this behavior is causing you harm. It also wants you to change, but for very different reasons.

- Put your hands over your heart or another soothing place, feeling their warmth. Now reflect again on the behavior you're struggling with. Begin to repeat the following phrases that capture the essence of your inner compassionate voice:

    - "I love you and I don't want you to suffer."

    - Or if it feels more authentic, say something like "I deeply care about you, and that's why I'd like to help you make a change." Or "I'm here for you and will support you."

- When you're ready, begin to write a message to yourself in the voice of your inner compassionate self. Write freely and spontaneously, addressing the behavior you would like to change. What emerges from the deep feeling and wish "I love you and don't want you to suffer"? What do you need to hear to make a change? Or if it's a struggle to find words, try writing down the words that would flow from your loving heart when speaking to a dear friend who was struggling with the same issue as you.

REFLECTION

What was that exercise like for you? Could you identify the voice of inner criticism?

Did you find any way your critical voice was trying to help you? Did it make sense to thank the inner critic for its efforts?

What was the impact of saying the words "I love you and don't want you to suffer"? Could you get in touch with your inner compassionate voice? Were you able to write from this perspective?

If you found some words that came from your inner compassionate self, let yourself *savor* the feeling of being supported. If you had *difficulty* finding words of kindness, that's okay too. It takes some time. The important thing is that we set our intention to be more self-compassionate, and eventually new habits will form.

This is a powerful exercise for many people. The revelation that our inner critic is actually trying to help us allows us to stop judging ourselves for judging ourselves. Once we see that the inner critic is trying to keep us safe by screaming "Danger! Danger!" and we validate those efforts and thank the critic for its good intentions, the critic usually relaxes and makes space for another voice to emerge—the voice of our inner compassionate self. (For more on this approach, readers might wish to explore the internal family systems model of Richard Schwartz.)

Many people find it especially surprising that our inner critic and our inner compassionate self are often seeking the same behavior change—the message simply has a very different quality or tone. As a humorous aside, an MSC participant once told us, "It's amazing. My inner critic used to always scream at me 'You bitch!' And my inner compassionate self just said, 'Whoa, Tiger . . . '"

Some readers might experience backdraft after this exercise. If you do, refer to Chapter 8 for guidance about how to work with backdraft, such as labeling the emotion, taking a walk and feeling the soles of your feet, or engaging in ordinary, pleasant activities. Sometimes the most compassionate thing we can do for ourselves is to have a chat with friends or simply to disengage from self-compassion practice for a while.

INFORMAL PRACTICE
Compassionate Letter to Myself

You can continue listening to your compassionate voice by writing a letter to yourself whenever you struggle or feel inadequate or when you want to help motivate yourself to make a change. There are three main ways you can write the letter:

- Think of an imaginary friend who is unconditionally wise, loving, and compassionate and write a letter to yourself *from the perspective of your friend.*

- Write a letter *as if you were talking to a dearly beloved friend* who was struggling with the same concerns as you.

- Write a letter from the compassionate part of yourself to the part of yourself that is struggling.

After writing the letter, you can put it down for a while and then read it later, letting the words soothe and comfort you when you need it most.

It can take a while to feel comfortable writing to yourself in the voice of a good friend, but it definitely gets easier with practice. This is a sample letter that Karen, an up-and-coming graphic designer, wrote to herself about not spending the time she'd like with her two children, ages 8 and 13. She wrote it as if it were coming from her best friend, with whom she is very close.

Dearest Karen, I know you feel bad about not spending enough time with your kids. You had to miss little Sophie's ballet rehearsal, and Ben had to microwave their dinner twice last week when you were held up at work. But please don't beat yourself up about it. It hurts me when you do that. You're a good mom, and the time you spend with your kids is real quality time. It's been so tough trying to balance your career with your family life. You need to give yourself a break. You're doing the best you can, and the way I see it you're doing incredibly well. Your kids love you deeply. I love you deeply.

I know you'd like to not work such late hours so that you can spend more time with Sophie and Ben. Maybe you can talk to your boss about it and tell him your concerns. You've been with the company seven years now and proven yourself. You're allowed to ask for what you need. The worst that can happen is he says no. And even if things don't change, you're a loving mom. Please don't forget that.

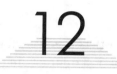

Self-Compassion and Our Bodies

Although we struggle to feel good enough in many areas of our lives, an area of particular challenge is our bodies. Our sense of self is closely identified with the body, so our physical appearance has a large impact on how we feel about ourselves. Body image may be particularly important for women because the standards of female beauty are so high. Increasingly, women are turning to surgery ("getting a little work done") to look like those perfect models in the magazines. Yet try as they might, most women will certainly fall short of the ideal—even the models' photos are airbrushed!

Men tend to be more satisfied than women by the way they look, but they still have trouble accepting their bodies—"Am I fit enough, slim enough, manly enough?" A man's preoccupation may lie more in how the body performs, such as how strong he may be, or how skilled in sports, or his sexual prowess.

No matter what challenges we face, both men and women are likely to see their bodies as adversaries rather than as friends. Rather than saying "Ughh!" when the body doesn't look or behave the way we imagine it should, a self-compassionate response to the body might be "Awwww." In other words, can we recognize how hard the body tries to persevere despite poor diet, lack of sleep, insufficient exercise, and aging, and feel tenderness toward the body? That's a big deal for both sexes.

Jillian was 52 and "past her prime." While she had always struggled with her weight and never thought her body was attractive enough, her struggle only intensified when she hit middle age. She turned her nose up in disgust every time she caught a glimpse of herself in the mirror, and she was filled with feelings of inadequacy. Jillian had bags under her eyes and saddle bags on her thighs. In fact, she was starting to feel "baggy" all over. She tried to find solace in peanut butter and chocolate ice cream, but the relief was short-lived, to say the least. Jillian tried not to obsess about her body but couldn't help it. She never really felt comfortable with her appearance because she didn't feel good enough on the inside.

Fortunately, self-compassion offers a powerful antidote to body dissatisfaction. Research shows that just a brief period of practicing self-compassion can help us feel less body shame, reduce the degree to which our feelings of self-worth are contingent on physical appearance, and help us appreciate our bodies as they are.

When we treat ourselves with kindness, warmth, and acceptance—even when the image we see in the mirror isn't perfect—we realize that we are so much more than this image. We begin to see that our worth stems from being a human being who tries to be happy and often gets it wrong, but keeps trying anyway. Instead of identifying with the body as the definition of who we are, we can see the bigger picture, realizing that our inner resources and inner beauty are most important. We can stop to appreciate the amazing gift of life our body provides us, feeling our aliveness deep within our being. With self-compassion we can celebrate our bodies for what they still do for us, rather than merely how they look, and begin to end the madness.

After she learned to practice self-compassion, Jillian's relationship with herself and her body started to change. She realized that she wanted other people to think she was beautiful so that she would feel loved and accepted, but that it was really up to her to love and accept herself. Yes, Jillian was growing a bit stout with age, but with age was coming wisdom and a newfound sense of her strengths—of what she had to give to the world. She wasn't perfect on the inside or outside, but she began to appreciate how her flaws made her real and authentic, that they were signs of her own precious humanity. Jillian wasn't a robot or a Stepford wife—she was flesh and blood and pulsed with life-giving energy.

As Jillian changed her relationship to herself, her relationship to food also changed. She no longer needed to stuff herself with food to feel full emotionally. She could enjoy her food but stop when her body said enough. And the biggest shift was that Jillian finally started to feel that she was enough, *that being human was enough, and could finally start to love and accept herself for who she was.*

EXERCISE
Embracing Our Bodies with Self-Compassion

Having compassion for physical imperfection is difficult in a competitive culture that is obsessed with the body. We are surrounded by unrealistic media images, making it almost impossible not to be dissatisfied with how we look or perform. Our only option is to accept the fact that we aren't perfect, do the best we can, and love ourselves anyway. This exercise is designed to help you accept yourself as you are and to embrace your imperfection with the three elements of self-compassion.

- Start by using the space below to make a kind but honest assessment of your body. See if you can be mindful of what is true—the good and the bad. First list all the features of your body that you like. Maybe you're in good health and have an attractive smile. Don't overlook things that may not normally factor into your self-image: the fact that you have strong hands or that your digestive system functions well (not to be taken for granted!). Let yourself fully acknowledge and appreciate the aspects of your body that you're happy with.

- Now, list all the features of your body that you don't like so well. Maybe your skin is blemished, or you have belly rolls, or you cannot run as far and fast as you could when you were younger. As you do this, feelings of discomfort may arise, and see if you can acknowledge this too. "It's hard to see how my jawline is slackening; this is difficult for me." See if you can stay with these feelings, really acknowledging and accepting your imperfections without running away with an exaggerated story line of inadequacy. Try to make a balanced assessment of your "flaws." Is the fact that your hair is turning gray really such a problem? Are those extra ten pounds really an issue in terms of feeling good and healthy in your body? Don't try to minimize your imperfections, but don't blow them out of proportion either.

■ Next, see if you can acknowledge the common humanity in what you are feeling. Do you think others feel the same way you do? Is there a way in which body dissatisfaction is part of being human in today's society?

■ Finally, try giving yourself some kindness and compassion for the difficult emotions you are experiencing. How might you soothe and comfort yourself in this moment? Can you bring some acceptance to yourself, allowing yourself to be exactly as you are, flaws and all? If you are struggling to come up with words of kindness, you could imagine what you might say to a beloved friend who was struggling with these same sorts of body image issues. What type of warmth and support might you offer this friend to let him know that you care? Now try offering these words to yourself.

REFLECTION

What was it like to mindfully acknowledge those aspects of your body that you like and that you don't like? Did anything shift when you remembered common humanity? Were you able to bring kindness to yourself in the midst of your struggle?

This can be a challenging exercise because for most of us our self-esteem is so dependent on our physical appearance. If the exercise brought up difficult emotions, try to be kind to yourself for the pain of body dissatisfaction, perhaps by using Soothing Touch or taking a Self-Compassion Break (see Chapter 4).

Also, some people have specific behavioral goals, such as exercising more or eating a healthier diet, but they worry that by being compassionate with themselves they'll lose their motivation to change. Remember we can love and accept ourselves as we are, and at the same time encourage ourselves to adopt new behaviors that will make us healthier and happier.

MEDITATION

Compassionate Body Scan

In this meditation, we will be bringing warmhearted attention to each part of the body in a variety of ways, moving from one part to another, practicing how to be with each part of the body in a kind and compassionate way. We will be inclining our awareness toward the body with curiosity and tenderness, perhaps as you might incline toward a young child.

If you feel ease and well-being in a particular body part, you can invite some gratitude or appreciation to arise within you toward that part of your body. If you have judgments or unpleasant sensations regarding a body part, perhaps you can let your heart soften in sympathy for the struggle, maybe also place a hand on that part of your body as a gesture of compassion and support and imagine warmth and kindness flowing through your hand and fingers into your body.

And if any area of your body is too difficult to stay with, feel free to move your attention to another body part for a while, especially a body part that is emotionally or physically neutral, allowing this meditation to be as comfortable as possible.

Stay in touch with what you need, moment to moment.

Readers can familiarize themselves with the instructions and then close their eyes and move their awareness compassionately through the body. For beginners, it will be much easier to use a guided recording (see the end of the Contents for information).

- Find a comfortable position, resting on your back with your hands about six inches from your sides and your feet shoulder width apart. Then place one or two hands over your heart (or another soothing place), doing this as a reminder to bring loving, connected presence to your body throughout this exercise. Feel the warmth and gentle touch of your hands. Take three slow, relaxing breaths and then return your arms to your sides, if you like.

- Start with the *toes on your left foot,* and begin to notice if there are any sensations in your toes. Are your toes warm or cool, dry or moist? Just feel the sensations in your toes—ease, discomfort, or perhaps nothing at all—and let each sensation be just as it is. If your toes feel good, perhaps give your toes a wiggle and a smile of appreciation.

- Then move to the *sole* of your left foot. Can you detect any sensations there? Your feet have such a small surface area, yet they hold up your entire body all day long. They work so hard. Feel free to send your left sole a bit of gratitude if that feels right. If there is any discomfort, open to it in a tender way.

- Now sense your *whole foot.* If your foot feels comfortable, you can also extend gratitude for the discomfort that you *don't* have. If there *is* any discomfort, allow that area to soften as if it were wrapped in a warm towel. If you like, validate your discomfort with kind words, such as "There's a little discomfort there; it's okay for now."

- Gradually move your attention up your leg, one part at a time, noticing whatever body sensations are present, send some appreciation if the part feels fine, and send compassion if there is any discomfort. Still focusing on your left side, move slowly though the body, to your . . .

  ○ Ankle
  ○ Shin and calf
  ○ Knee

- When you notice your mind has wandered, as it always will, just return to the sensations in the part of your body you were attending to.

- You might also wish to add some words of kindness or compassion, such as "May my [knees] be at ease. May they be well." Then return your attention to the simple sensations in each body part.

- Allow this entire process to be exploratory, even playful, gently working your way through your body. Moving on to your . . .
  - Thigh
  - Hip

- If you feel uneasy or judgmental about a particular body part, try putting a hand over your heart and gently breathing, imagining that kindness and compassion are flowing through your fingers into your body.

- Or if you feel ease, offer an inner smile of appreciation, if that feels right to you.

- Now bring loving awareness to your *entire left leg*, making room for whatever you may be sensing or feeling.

- And moving on to the *right leg*, to your . . .
  - Right toes
  - Right sole
  - Right foot
  - Ankle
  - Shin and calf
  - Knee

- Feel free to skip any part of the body if too much physical or emotional discomfort arises. Now on to your . . .
  - Thigh
  - Hip
  - Entire right leg

- Now bring your awareness to your *pelvic area*—the strong bones that support your legs and also the soft tissue in your pelvic area. Perhaps feeling your buttocks on the floor or on the chair—large muscles that help you climb stairs and also allow you to sit softly and comfortably.

- And now your *lower back*—a lot of stress is stored in the lower back. If you notice any discomfort or tension, you might imagine your muscles relaxing, melting with tenderness.

- Feel free to shift your posture a little if an adjustment will make you more comfortable.

- And then your *upper back*.

- And now moving your attention to the front of your body, to your *abdomen*. Your abdomen is a very complicated part of the body with many organs and body functions. Perhaps sending some gratitude to this part of the body. If you have judgments about your belly, see if you can say some words of kindness and acceptance.

- Then moving up to your chest. The center of your breathing, also your heart center. This place is the source of love and compassion. Try to infuse your chest with awareness, appreciation, and acceptance. Perhaps put a gentle hand on the center of your chest, allowing yourself to feel whatever it is you're feeling right now.

- You should feel free to touch any part of the body as we go along, even gently stroking that part, whatever feels right to you.

- Continue to incline your awareness toward your body with the same quality of warmth you might have toward a young child, feeling the sensations in your . . .

  ○ Left shoulder
  ○ Left upper arm
  ○ Elbow

- Bring tender awareness to each part of your body. Your . . .

  ○ Left lower arm
  ○ Wrist
  ○ Hand
  ○ Fingers

- Feel free to wiggle your fingers, if you like, savoring the sensations that arise when you move your fingers. Your hands are uniquely designed to hold and manipulate fine objects, and are very sensitive to touch.

- And now scan your whole left arm and hand with loving and compassionate awareness.

- And moving to your right side, to your . . .

  ○ Right shoulder
  ○ Right upper arm
  ○ Elbow
  ○ Lower arm
  ○ Wrist
  ○ Hand
  ○ Fingers
  ○ Whole right arm and hand

- And now proceed with awareness toward the head, beginning with the *neck*. If you like, touch your neck with your hand, remembering how the neck supports your head throughout the day, how it is a conduit for blood to the brain and air to the body. Offer appreciation and kindness to your neck—either mentally or with physical touch—if your neck feels good, or sending compassion if there is any tension or discomfort there.

- Finally, moving on to your *head,* beginning with the back of the head, the hard surface that protects your brain. If you like, gently touch the back of your head with your hand or simply touch it with loving awareness.

- And then your *ears*—those sensitive organs of perception that tell us so much about our world. If you are glad you have the capacity to hear, allow appreciation to arise in your heart. If you are worried about your hearing, perhaps put a hand over your heart and give yourself some compassion.

- And then offer the same loving or compassionate awareness to your other organs of perception, such as your . . .
  - ○ Eyes
  - ○ Nose
  - ○ Lips
- Don't forget to recognize your *cheeks, jaw,* and *chin* for how they help you eat and speak and smile.
- And finally, your *forehead* and the *crown of your head* and, underneath . . . your *brain.* Your tender brain is comprised of billions of nerve cells that are communicating with each other all the time to help you make sense of this marvelous world we live in. If you like, say "thank you" to your brain for working 24/7 on your behalf.
- When you have finished giving kind and compassionate attention to your whole body, try offering your body a final shower—head to toe—of appreciation, compassion, and respect.
- And then gently open your eyes.

REFLECTION

What was this meditation like for you? What did you notice? Was it easier to feel sensations in some parts of your body than others?

Were you able to have compassion for those body parts that you judged or that felt uncomfortable? Did you try putting a soothing hand there? What was it like to send appreciation to your body?

Try not to criticize yourself if your attention wandered during this meditation, or if you found it frustrating, or even boring. Some people are not very interested in their bodies, or they prefer not to linger in their bodies for very long. Other people have the experience of being finally "home" when they practice the body scan. Everybody is different. Allow yourself to have whatever experience you had and allow yourself to be just as you are, with great kindness. That's mindfulness and self-compassion.

13

Stages of Progress

Self-compassion practice typically goes through three stages:

- Striving
- Disillusionment
- Radical acceptance

When we first start to practice being kinder to ourselves, we are likely to bring the same attitude to the process that we bring to other areas of our lives—we *strive* to get it right. And when we actually *experience* self-compassion, we may feel considerable relief and even greater enthusiasm for the practice. This early stage of self-compassion practice can be like the early stage of any love relationship—infatuation. We may be delighted by our newfound happiness and become attached to the experience and the person who brings it. Similarly, when we realize that we can meet our *own* needs, at least partially, that wonderful discovery may feel like falling in love. It can be quite uplifting.

> The first stage of learning self-compassion can feel like falling in love.

When Jonathan first used the Self-Compassion Break (see Chapter 4), he couldn't believe how powerful it was. He was thinking about a very stressful situation at work, and the brief practice instantly transformed his stress into a state of peace and calm. "You mean all I have to do is be mindful of my pain, acknowledge my shared humanity, and be kind to myself?" he thought. "This is amazing!"

But as with all new relationships, the shine eventually starts to wear off. For example, we may put our hands over our hearts, hoping to feel the safety and connection that we initially experienced, and nothing happens. Darn! So we move into the next stage of practice—*disillusionment*. When self-compassion begins to fail us, we think it's just one more thing we can't do right.

As a meditation teacher once said, "All techniques are destined to fail." Why? Because whenever our practice becomes a "technique" designed to manipulate our moment-to-moment experience—to make us feel better and make the pain go away—it becomes a hidden form of resistance. And we know how well resistance works!

> *When Jonathan got into a big argument with his teenage son and felt angry and frustrated, he thought he knew what to do to calm himself . . . the Self-Compassion Break! Unfortunately, that didn't work, so Jonathan tried Soothing Touch (see Chapter 4). That didn't work either. Feeling as if he were abandoned by a trusted friend, Jonathan became disheartened. "I thought I had it all figured out, but I still feel as miserable as ever. I must be really bad at self-compassion."*

When the despair of disillusionment brings us to our knees and we surrender in hopelessness, progress finally begins. Progress really means dropping the idea of progress. We stop striving to get somewhere, to achieve the goal of being good at self-compassion, of making the pain go away, and start to refine our intention. Rather than being attached to the outcome of self-compassion practice, we begin to do it for its own sake. We enter the stage of *radical acceptance,* which is best captured by the paradox mentioned in Chapter 7:

When we struggle, we give ourselves compassion not to feel better but *because* we feel bad.

In other words, in a moment of struggle, we don't practice to be free of our pain—we practice compassion because sometimes it's hard to be a human being. Radical acceptance is like a parent comforting a child who has the 48-hour flu. The parent doesn't care for the child to try to drive the flu away—the flu is going to leave in its own time. But because the child has a fever and feels bad, the parent comforts her as a natural response to suffering while the process of healing occurs.

It's like this when we try to comfort ourselves, too. When we fully accept the reality that we are imperfect human beings, prone to making mistakes and struggling, our hearts naturally begin to soften. We still feel pain, but we also feel the love *holding* the pain, and it's more bearable. This response is "radical" because it runs counter to how we normally relate to our pain, and the transformation can be equally radical.

> *After talking to a meditation teacher, Jonathan realized that the intention behind his self-compassion practice had unconsciously shifted. He had been so relieved that self-compassion made him feel better that he fell into the tendency*

to use it to make the pain go away when he felt bad. Eventually Jonathan real-ized that his life would never be pain-free. As this insight entered his heart, Jonathan noticed a quiet tenderness emerge whenever he found himself strug-gling. He even began to consider pain as a reminder to open his heart and that having an open heart was, after all, the thing he wanted most in life anyway.

As the meditation teacher Pema Chödrön says: "We can still be crazy after all these years. We can still be angry after all these years. We can still be timid or jeal-ous or full of feelings of unworthiness. The point is . . . not to try to throw ourselves away and become something better. It's about befriending who we are already."

The meditation teacher Rob Nairn puts it even more succinctly: "The goal of practice is to become a compassionate mess." That means fully human—often strug-gling, uncertain, confused—with great compassion. And the beautiful thing is that this is actually an achievable goal. No matter how precipitously we may fall, how gut-wrenching our pain, how imperfect our lives or personalities may be, we can still be mindful of our suffering, remember our common humanity, and be kind to ourselves.

The stages of progress do not always proceed in a linear, sequential fashion. They are more like a spiral going round and round, or sometimes we bounce back and forth from one stage to another. Over time, however, periods of striving and dis-illusionment become shorter and radical acceptance accompanies us more and more through the vicissitudes of our lives. We start to trust that no matter what happens, we can still hold ourselves in the embrace of loving, connected presence.

 EXERCISE

Where Am I in My Self-Compassion Practice?

Use the spaces provided to record the thoughts that come up when you con-sider the following three questions:

- Remembering that we cycle through the stages of progress in our self-compassion practice, take a moment to reflect on what part of the cycle you might be in right now—striving, disillusionment, or radical acceptance?

- If you are struggling in some areas of your practice, is there any way you can reduce the struggle? Is there any experience that you would like to give a little more space, or let go of, or allow more fully?

- Is there any way you can bring compassion to yourself in the midst of your journey? Can you be gentle and patient as your practice unfolds, perhaps saying some words of kindness, understanding, support, or appreciation?

REFLECTION

As soon as people hear the term *progress,* they often think "the more progress the better." In other words, people may judge themselves for not being in the stage of radical acceptance. It's important to realize that self-compassion is a way of being, not a destination. Although we will have moments of radical acceptance, we will also have many moments of striving and disillusionment. These are all equally important aspects of the path. Therefore, if you are experiencing any judgment (positive or negative) about where you are in the stages of progress, see if you can also let go of the habit of self-evaluation and simply open to what is true for you in the moment, with a tender heart.

 INFORMAL PRACTICE
Being a Compassionate Mess

Whenever you find yourself using self-compassion to try to make the pain go away or to become a "better person," try shifting your focus away from this subtle form of resistance and practice compassion simply because we're all imperfect human beings living an imperfect life. And life is hard. In other words, practice being a "compassionate mess." This practice can be done in the midst of daily life whenever you are struggling.

- Think of a situation in your life that is causing you emotional pain because you feel inadequate in some way. Perhaps you did something you regret or failed at something important to you. Choose a problem in the mild-to-moderate range, not a big problem, as we want to build the resource of self-compassion gradually.

- Can you feel discomfort in your body as you bring this situation to mind? If not, choose a slightly more difficult situation, but if you are feeling a lot of discomfort, choose a less difficult situation.

- As you are feeling emotional discomfort, see if you can fully accept that pain, allowing your heart to melt as you hold these difficult feelings, to soothe and care for yourself *because* it's so difficult. Can you accompany yourself through this moment with your own loving, connected presence?

- Take two or three deep breaths and close your eyes for a few moments to settle and center yourself. Put your hands on your heart or use some other soothing touch as a gesture of support and self-kindness.

- Try speaking to yourself (out loud or silently), using warm, supportive, compassionate language. For example:
  - "I'm so sorry you're feeling so badly about yourself right now, but these feelings won't last forever. I'm here for you; it's going to be okay."

- "The pain of failure is almost overwhelming. I can't make it go away, but I will try to be with it with courage, patience, and an open heart."

- Can you allow yourself to be as you are—fully human? Can you begin to let go of striving for perfection and acknowledge that you are doing the best you can? Try speaking to yourself using language that acknowledges your imperfection but that also gives a sense of unconditional acceptance—language you might use with a friend or someone you really cared about. For example:

  - "It's okay to be a compassionate mess, to be imperfect."

  - "Wow, I really screwed up. I wish I hadn't, but I did. It's really tough to feel this way. There's nothing I can do to change the fact that I'm an imperfect human being who sometimes gets it wrong. May I try to accept myself with understanding and kindness."

REFLECTION

It's natural to resist letting go of striving to get it right or accepting our imperfection. We want to feel safe, and making mistakes makes us feel unsafe. But we don't need to add insult to injury by judging ourselves for wanting to be other than we are. We just need to realize how this struggle may be causing us unnecessary suffering, explore whether we can at least *begin* to accept ourselves and our human flaws, and see what happens.

14

Living Deeply

The fundamental self-compassion question is "What do I need?" But we can't really give ourselves what we need if we don't know what we value most in our lives. These are our core values, those deeply held ideals that guide us and give meaning to our lives. Both needs and values seem to reflect something essential in human nature. Needs are more commonly associated with physical and emotional survival, such as the need for health and safety, or for love and connection, whereas values tend to have an element of choice, such as the choice to focus on social justice or creative pursuits.

> *Identifying your core values can help you give yourself what you really need.*

Our struggles in life depend a great deal on our core values. For example, if you value free time and new adventures, not getting a promotion that would have required working extra hours may be a blessing; but if you value providing for your family, being passed over for a promotion could be devastating.

There is a difference between *goals* and *core values*:

Goals can be *achieved*.	Core values still guide us even after we achieve our goals.
Goals are *destinations*.	Core values are *directions*.
Goals are something we *do*.	Core values are something we *are*.
Goals are *set*.	Core values are *discovered*.
Goals often come from outside.	Core values come from deep within.

Examples of core values are compassion, generosity, honesty, and service. Many of our core values are relational values—how we want to be treated and to treat others—but others are more personal, such as freedom, spiritual growth, exploration, or artistic expression.

Mark worked at a corporate law firm, drove a Lexus, and was, to the outside world, a success. His parents always expected him to be a doctor or a lawyer, but when he finally made partner he realized something was missing. He wasn't happy and didn't know how he had ended up living a life that was so far from what he wanted. Mark loved writing and would rather be crafting a novel than crafting lawsuits against copyright infringers. While he often dreamed of leaving his firm to become a fiction writer, he was afraid of his parents' disapproval if he did. Even more than that, he was terrified of failure, afraid of what would happen if he couldn't make a living as an author.

When we are not living in alignment with our core values, we suffer. An important act of self-compassion, therefore, is to identify our values, figure out whether we are living in accord with them, and try to give ourselves what we need. If we really care about our own happiness and want to alleviate our own suffering—in other words, if we have self-compassion—we will typically find the inner resources to live more in touch with our values and to live a deeper and more meaningful life.

Mark eventually sank into a depression and started seeing a therapist, who told him about self-compassion. Mark realized that if he was going to be a better friend to himself, he needed to spend time doing activities that he genuinely enjoyed. Mark was an early riser, so he began setting aside an hour every morning to work on a story that had been percolating in his mind for the past five years. This small change, which Mark called "first things first," made him feel happier and more energetic, and Mark discovered that his day at the office became less onerous. He joined a writing group that met after work, made some like-minded friends, started going to readings at a local bookstore, and generally felt that his life was getting on the right track. The internal pressure that Mark felt to change his career subsided, at least for now.

 EXERCISE

Discovering Our Core Values

Use the space provided to do this written reflection exercise.

- Imagine that you are in your elderly years. You're sitting in a lovely garden as you contemplate your life. Looking back, you feel a deep sense of satisfaction, joy, and contentment. Even though life hasn't always been easy, you managed to stay true to yourself to the best of your ability. Which core values did you live by that gave your life meaning? For example, spending time in nature, travel and adventure, or service to others. Please write down your core values.

- Now write down any ways you feel you are *not living in accord with your core values,* or ways in which your life feels out of balance with your values. For example, perhaps you are too busy to spend time in nature, even though connecting with nature is what you love most in life.

- If you have several values that you feel out of line with, choose one that is especially important to you and write it down.

- Of course, there are often obstacles that prevent us from living in accord with our core values. Some of these may be *external obstacles,* like not having enough money or time. For instance, maybe your job is so time-consuming that you don't have much time to spend in nature. If there are any external obstacles, write them down.

- There may also be some *internal obstacles* getting in the way of your living in accord with your core values. For instance, are you afraid of failure, do you doubt your abilities, or is your inner critic getting in the way? For instance, maybe you don't feel you are worthy of spending a carefree day in the woods. Write down any internal obstacles.

- Now consider whether *self-kindness and self-compassion could help you live in accord with your true values,* for example, by helping you overcome internal obstacles like your inner critic. Is there a way self-compassion could help you feel safe and confident enough to take new actions, or risk failure, or stop doing things that are a waste of your time? Or is there some way you can express your values in your life that you haven't thought of before? For example, get a job with a more flexible schedule so you can go camping more often?

- Finally, if there are *insurmountable obstacles* to living in accord with your values, can you give yourself compassion for that hardship? That is, not abandon your values in spite of the conditions? And if the insurmountable problem is that you are *imperfect*, as all human beings are, can you forgive yourself for that, too?

REFLECTION

What was this exercise like for you? Did you encounter anything unexpected?

Some people struggle to identify their core values when they do this exercise. It may be that we have been living our lives so intensely that we haven't even paused long enough to consider what values are deeply meaningful to us. In this case, self-compassion comes in the form of simply asking the question "What do I care about?" Are your values truly your own, or are they the values that others have told you that you *should* have?

Other people might be clear about their core values but are disappointed that they aren't living in accord with them. While it is useful to consider whether self-compassion can help us let go of things that get in our way, it's equally important to recognize that, try as we might, sometimes we just can't live in accord with our core values. If this is the case for you, see if you can accept that living a human life is complicated, all the while keeping the flame of your deepest desires burning in your heart. You may discover that a small expression of a core value can make a big difference in your life.

INFORMAL PRACTICE
Living with a Vow

Often our feelings of dissatisfaction, frustration, and anxiety arise out of an awareness that we are not living in accord with our core values. When we discover that we're "in the wrong place, at the wrong time, doing the wrong thing, with the wrong people," it's time to remember our core values.

A core value can be made into a vow to help us remember. *What is a vow?*

- A vow is an *aspiration* to which we can continually reorient ourselves when we've gone astray in our lives.

- A vow *anchors* our life in what matters most. It is not a binding contract.

- A vow *functions like the breath* in breath meditation—a safe place to return when we're lost and adrift in our daily lives.

We need to be very compassionate with ourselves when we notice we've strayed—no shame or self-recrimination—and then refocus on our core values.

Select an important core value you discovered from the last exercise that you would like to manifest for the rest of your life.

Now try writing it in the form of a vow: "May I . . ." or "I vow to . . . as best I can."

Close your eyes and repeat your vow silently several times.

REFLECTION

Were you able to create a vow that was meaningful? How did it feel to set your intention in this way?

Many people find that saying a vow each day helps keep them on track, like setting a GPS to find your way home. If you like, before you get out of bed in the morning, you can put your hand on your heart and say your vow a few times and then get up. You can do the same before you go to sleep. Sometimes it helps to have a little ritual, such as lighting a candle when you make your vow.

 EXERCISE
Silver Linings

Another important aspect of living deeply is learning from struggles and challenges in our lives. While most of us are afraid of hardship and failure, it's often these experiences that teach us lessons we wouldn't have learned otherwise. Thich Nhat Hanh says, "No mud, no lotus." In other words, without being rooted in the muck of life, we wouldn't be able to blossom into our full potential. Challenges can force us to go deep inside and discover resources and insights we didn't know we had. The saying "Every cloud has a silver lining" refers to this truth. One of the gifts of self-compassion is that it allows us to be present with our suffering without being overwhelmed, giving us the support needed for growth and discovery to occur.

> *Growing into our full potential starts with being rooted in the mud.*

Before starting this exercise, you may want to take two or three deep breaths and close your eyes for a few moments to settle and center yourself. Try putting your hands over your heart or use some other soothing touch as a gesture of support and kindness.

- Think of a past struggle in your own life that seemed very difficult or even impossible to bear at the time and that, looking back, taught you an important lesson. Choose an event that is far enough in the past that it is clearly resolved and you learned what you needed to learn. What was the situation? Please write it down.

- What deeper lesson did the challenge or crisis teach you that you probably would never have learned otherwise? Write that down, too.

- As a thought experiment, consider whether there is a *current* difficulty in your life that might also have a silver lining. And if so, what *hidden lesson* might be contained in your current dilemma?

- How might the practice of self-compassion help you feel safe and strong in this situation, so that you can learn what you need to learn?

REFLECTION

What was your experience of this exercise? Were you able to find a potential silver lining in a current difficulty or consider how self-compassion might help you do so?

Sometimes difficult situations have no silver lining, and it's a significant achievement simply to have survived. If that is the case for you, take a moment to appreciate your resilience.

Remembering the learning that comes through struggle helps us reframe our suffering in a more positive light. Of course, this process doesn't mean denying the difficulty. If you had a hard time seeing the silver lining of a current situation, this is only natural, and it shouldn't be forced. Simply opening up to the possibility that struggle contains growth can help us hold things a bit more lightly.

15

Being There for Others
without Losing Ourselves

One way that self-compassion transforms our lives is by allowing us to give to others without losing ourselves. When we are present for others while they're experiencing pain, we feel the pain inside us—literally. Some scientists have posited a special type of neuron dedicated to perceiving in our own bodies what others are experiencing, called *mirror neurons*. There are also areas in the brain dedicated to evaluating social situations and resonating with the emotions of others. This type of empathic resonance often happens at a preverbal, visceral level.

Empathic resonance is evolutionarily adaptive because it allows us to cooperate with one another to better raise our young and defend ourselves against danger. We're hardwired for social interaction. Although empathy is usually a good thing, it can also be a problem, because when we're resonating with others in pain—especially with people we know well—we feel their pain as our own. Sometimes empathic distress can feel overwhelming. When that happens, we may try various maneuvers to avoid and reduce *our* suffering, such as tuning out the other person or taking the elevator up into our heads and trying to fix the problem. (For more on this topic, see Chapters 18 and 19.)

Have you ever wondered why, when you tried to tell someone about a struggle you were having, the listener immediately jumped in with advice on how to fix it without really listening to your story? Or have *you* ever done this to someone else? This reaction is quite common, but why do we do it? One reason is that it's uncomfortable to be in the presence of someone else's pain because we are cofeeling their pain. Empathic distress can also bring up fears or uncomfortable memories from our own lives.

Maria considered herself the sensitive type, always wanting to help others. One day her close friend Ayesha asked to go out for a cup of coffee. In tears, Ayesha told Maria about a very recent breakup with her long-term boyfriend. Instead of letting Ayesha tell her story, however, Maria found she kept interrupting her friend, reminding Ayesha it was going to be all right and that she would find someone new. Finally, in exasperation, Ayesha blurted out, "Why can't you just listen *to me? I'm grieving, and I need to let it out. Maybe I will be all right* someday, *but I'm not okay now. I need you to be here for me now!" Visibly upset, Ayesha got up and left the table.*

Although Maria was trying to help, her approach just made things worse. Those of us who are problem solvers may feel particularly inclined to "fix" the pain of others. Although well intentioned, interrupting others without fully listening and validating their pain can break the emotional connection with the speaker. The speaker was probably hoping, consciously or unconsciously, to receive compassion. Compassion is a resource that enables someone to hold pain without immediately having to make it go away. It also allows us to care for the *person* who is experiencing the pain with great tenderness.

How do we maintain emotional connection with others in pain? First, we need to stay in connection with *ourselves*—we need to be aware of our own empathic distress and be compassionate with ourselves. When we are open and accepting of our ongoing reactions to the speaker and we have compassion for how difficult it is to listen sometimes, we can allow the other person to speak without needing to interrupt them or distract ourselves during the conversation.

> *Sustaining empathy for others begins with compassion for ourselves.*

After Ayesha left, and Maria had a chance to collect her thoughts, Maria realized how distressing it was to see her friend so upset. She just wanted to stop Ayesha's pain by offering helpful counsel, which obviously backfired because Ayesha didn't get the compassionate ear she so desperately needed. Furthermore, Maria's sense of being overwhelmed was amplified by memories of a similar breakup of her own one year earlier.

Maria loved her friend very much, so she went by her house later that evening to apologize and ask to talk some more. This time, as Ayesha related her story, Maria practiced Compassionate Listening (see page 113). Whenever Maria felt uncomfortable, she offered herself a long, comforting inbreath. Maria soon discovered it was much easier to listen to Ayesha. She was happy and relieved that she could really be there for her friend after all—and also be there for herself.

MEDITATION
Giving and Receiving Compassion

This meditation builds on two previous meditations—Affectionate Breathing (Chapter 6) and Loving-Kindness for Ourselves (Chapter 10)—and involves both breath awareness and the intentional cultivation of kindness and compassion. It is the third core meditation of the MSC course. We can breathe in for ourselves and out for others. Breathing out expands the meditation to include others, and breathing in helps us remember to be self-compassionate. (You can find a guided recording of this meditation online; see the end of the Contents for information.)

> *What do you need to feel safe and comfortable with others?*

- Sit comfortably, close your eyes, and if you like, put a hand over your heart or another soothing place as a reminder to bring not just awareness but *loving* awareness to your experience and to yourself.

Savoring the Breath

- Take a few deep, relaxing breaths, noticing how your breath nourishes your body as you inhale and soothes your body as you exhale.

- Now let your breath find its own natural rhythm. Continue feeling the sensation of breathing in and breathing out. If you like, allow yourself to be gently rocked and caressed by the rhythm of your breathing.

Warming Up Awareness

- Now focus your attention on your *inbreath,* letting yourself savor the sensation of breathing in, noticing how your inbreath nourishes your body, breath after breath . . . and then release your breath.

- As you breathe, begin to breathe in kindness and compassion for yourself. Just feel the quality of kindness and compassion as you breathe in, or if you prefer, letting a word or image ride on your inbreath.

- Now shift your focus to your *outbreath,* feeling your body breathe out, feeling the ease of exhalation.

- Please call to mind *someone whom you love* or *someone who is struggling and needs compassion.* Visualize that person clearly in your mind.

- Begin directing your outbreath to this person, offering the ease of breathing out.

- If you wish, send kindness and compassion to this person with each outbreath, one breath after another.

In for Me, Out for You

- Now focus on the sensation of breathing *both* in and out, savoring the sensation of breathing in and out.

- Begin breathing in for yourself and out for the other person. "In for me and out for you." "One for me and one for you."

- And as you breathe, draw kindness and compassion in for yourself and breathe kindness and compassion out for the other person.

- If you wish, you can focus a little more on yourself ("Two for me and one for you") or the other person ("One for me and three for you"), or just let it be an equal flow—whatever feels right in the moment.

- Let go of any unnecessary effort, allowing this meditation to be as easy as breathing.

- Allow your breath to flow in and out, like the gentle movement of the ocean— a limitless, boundless flow—flowing in and flowing out. Let yourself be a *part* of this limitless, boundless flow. An ocean of compassion.

- Gently open your eyes.

REFLECTION

What did you notice during this meditation? What did you feel? Was it easier to breathe in for yourself or out for the other? Were you able to adjust the flow when needed, focusing more on yourself or the other according to whose need was most salient?

It can be a great relief to give compassion to ourselves while we are being compassionate to others. Some people, however, don't like to focus on themselves at all, especially if the other person is in a great deal of pain. It's important to adjust the direction of our breathing so that it feels just right. Sometimes it may feel right to focus primarily on breathing out for the other, at other times primarily on breathing in for oneself. As long as everyone is included in the circle of compassion, a natural state of balance will eventually be found.

This meditation forms the basis of other practices designed to help us be there for others without losing ourselves and can be a wonderful part of your daily 30-minute practice.

INFORMAL PRACTICE
Compassionate Listening

This is a practice you can try next time you are listening to someone who is telling you a distressing story. It will help you maintain an emotional connection with the speaker and keep you from feeling overwhelmed.

Embodied Listening

- The first step is to *listen in an embodied way.* Listen with your whole body, letting yourself feel whatever sensations arise in your body, as well as paying attention with your eyes and your ears. And if it feels right to you, let yourself embody loving, connected presence (i.e., compassion). Let your body radiate this energy in both directions—toward yourself and also toward the speaker.

- As you listen, you will have many natural reactions. For example, you may find yourself emotionally hooked or overwhelmed by what you hear, you may become distracted by your own story as it relates to what you are hearing, or you may feel an urgent need to interrupt the speaker and "fix" the person's problem.

Giving and Receiving Compassion

- When you find your attention wandering off, that's when you can begin practicing Giving and Receiving Compassion informally, on the spot. Just focus on your breath for a while, breathing compassion in for yourself and out for the speaker. Breathing in for yourself will reconnect you with your body and breathing out will reconnect you with the speaker, allowing you to be present in the midst of the speaker's pain. Giving some attention to breathing out in this way may also satisfy your urge to help the speaker by fixing his problem (i.e., interrupting).

- Continue breathing compassion in and out until you can listen again in an embodied way. We don't want to focus *too much* on our breathing while listening because this type of multitasking can be distracting. Rather, compassionate breathing is simply a safety net to catch us when we become distracted, and it brings us back into loving, connected presence. In other words, being there for others without losing ourselves.

REFLECTION

After trying out this practice a few times while listening to others, reflect on how it impacts your experience of listening. If you find the breathing is getting in the way and distracting you, then perhaps lessen the amount of focus you put on the breath. But if you find you're still being overwhelmed by empathetic distress, or your urge to fix keeps getting the better of you, it may be wise to give more attention to being centered in your body and breathing in for yourself and out for the other as you listen. Experiment with it until you find a balance that works for you.

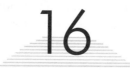

16

Meeting Difficult Emotions

Life isn't easy. It often brings challenging situations, and with them, difficult emotions such as anger, fear, worry, and grief. By a certain age, we learn that it doesn't help to run from our problems—we need to deal with them directly.

When we turn *toward* difficult emotions, however, even with mindfulness and self-compassion, our pain often increases at first and our natural instinct is to turn away. But if we are to heal, we must face them—the only way out is through. We must have the courage to be present with emotional pain if we are going to live healthy, authentic lives. Still, does this mean we need to face all our difficult emotions in their full intensity? Luckily, no. Someone once asked the meditation teacher Thich Nhat Hanh how much emotional distress we should allow into our practice. His answer was "Not much!"

Experiencing discomfort is necessary for self-compassion to arise, but we only need to *touch* emotional pain to cultivate compassion, and we can go slowly so we don't overwhelm ourselves. The art of self-compassion includes inclining *gradually* toward emotional discomfort when it arises.

> *We need to turn toward and be with our difficult emotions so we can heal.*

There are five stages of acceptance when meeting difficult emotions, and each successive stage corresponds to a gradual release of emotional resistance.

- *Resisting*: struggling against what comes—"Go away!
- *Exploring*: turning toward discomfort with curiosity—"What am I feeling?"
- *Tolerating*: safely enduring, holding steady—"I don't like this, but I can stand it."
- *Allowing*: letting feelings come and go—"It's okay, I can make space for this."
- *Befriending*: seeing value in difficult emotional experiences—"What can I learn from this?"

Readers can use the stages of acceptance as a guide for how to stay safe while engaging in the exercises in this book. It can be wise to back off from an exercise if it feels overwhelming, perhaps just remaining curious rather than opening fully to difficult emotions. Backing off in the service of safety may be the best lesson in self-compassion you could learn.

Ask yourself what you need—do you need to open or to close?

The resources of mindfulness and self-compassion help us work with difficult emotions without avoiding or resisting them, but without becoming overwhelmed either.

There are three particularly helpful strategies for working with difficult emotions:

- Labeling emotions
- Being aware of emotions in the body
- Soften–soothe–allow

The first two approaches are mindfulness based, and the third is more compassion oriented.

Labeling Emotions

"Name it and you tame it." Naming or labeling difficult emotions helps us disentangle, or "unstick," from them. Research shows that when we label difficult emotions, the amygdala—a brain structure that registers danger—becomes less active and is less likely to trigger a stress reaction in the body.

Naming a difficult emotion helps us not to get lost in it.

When we gently say, "This is anger" or "Fear is arising," we usually feel some emotional freedom—there is some space around the feeling. Instead of being lost in the emotion, we can recognize that we are having the emotion and therefore have more choice of how to respond.

Awareness of Emotions in the Body

"Feel it and you heal it." Emotions have mental and physical components—thoughts and bodily sensations. For example, when we're angry, we spend a lot of time in our minds justifying our point of view and planning what we will or should have said. We also feel physical tension in the abdomen as the body prepares for a fight.

It's more challenging to manage a difficult emotion by working with our thoughts because we're so easily swept away by them. It's a bit easier to work with the physical sensations of the emotion. Thoughts move so quickly that it's tough to hang on to them long enough to transform them. In contrast, the body is relatively slow moving. When we locate and anchor our emotions in the body—find the actual physical sensations of the emotion and hold them in mindful awareness—the difficult emotion often starts to change on its own.

When Keyla, a single mom, opened the bill from the college bookstore, she was shocked at the amount due. She had given her daughter, Dina, a credit card when she went off to college to buy textbooks and supplies but had no idea how expensive textbooks were these days. Keyla started getting upset, sweating and wringing her hands. She was already overdrawn at the bank after paying Dina's fall semester tuition. How was she going to pay for this? Would she have to take on more hours at work? But her doctor already said that her blood pressure was too high. Maybe ask her ex-husband for help? Fat chance! He had a new family and already said he was cutting off all support for Dina after she turned 18. The bastard. She would just have to call her daughter and tell her to return the books and, hopefully, borrow books from a friend. Or maybe Dina should just transfer to a cheaper community college?

Keyla knew she had to calm down and try to apply some of the mindfulness techniques she had been learning. She poured herself a cup of tea. Eventually she found the mental space to ask herself what she was feeling. "Fear? Wait, no . . . sadness!" It would be so sad to have to pull Dina out of the university she worked so hard to get into. Yes, the bill was higher than expected, but it wasn't going to ruin her. And her bonus was coming soon, which would help clear up the overdraft. Simply naming and validating her emotions enabled Keyla to get perspective on her situation and see things more clearly.

Next, Keyla tried to figure out where sadness resided in her body. It felt it mostly in her heart region, as a sense of hollowness. Also, some heaviness. As Keyla inclined her awareness toward the heart region of her body, the intensity of her sadness subsided still further.

Soften–Soothe–Allow

Difficult emotions are even more transitory—they pass through us more easily—when we establish a loving, accepting relationship to them. When our awareness has a fearful quality, we are less open to our emotions and can barely tolerate the experience. But when our awareness is tender and warm, we have the strength to feel what is happening within us and give ourselves what we need.

Soften–soothe–allow is a set of compassionate responses to difficult emotions we may find in the body. We can offer ourselves comfort in three ways:

- *Softening*—physical compassion
- *Soothing*—emotional compassion
- *Allowing*—mental compassion

The soften–soothe–allow technique adds compassion to the previous two mindfulness approaches. Rather than simply holding our difficult experience in spacious awareness, we warm up the embrace. Compassion provides an extra measure of emotional security, so we have the room to work with our emotions and learn from them.

When Keyla went to bed that evening, she had trouble falling asleep. She was still upset, so she tried using the soften–soothe–allow practice she had learned. First she went back to labeling what she was feeling—still mostly sadness, also tinged with fear—and felt the strong ache in her heart just like before. Then Keyla added a bit of compassion to the mix. She softened her body so she wasn't holding the sensation in her chest so tightly. Then she put a comforting hand over her heart and gently stroked her chest, making little circles in a gentle way, and spoke to herself as she might to a good friend. "I'm sorry about the financial strain you're going through right now, sweetheart. It's not fair. And, of course, it saddens you—you want the best for your daughter. Somehow we'll get through this."

Once Keyla gave herself understanding and support, her sadness didn't feel so overwhelming. She could allow it to be there, holding it with great tenderness. She also realized that there was something to learn from the situation. She often caused herself unnecessary suffering by assuming the worst-case scenario, and this was a major contributor to her high blood pressure. But she really didn't need to put herself through this torment. When Keyla held her fear and sadness (and herself!) in a courageous and kind manner, it didn't get the best of her. This insight gave Keyla confidence that she would be able to meet other challenges that lay ahead, particularly as a single mom.

INFORMAL PRACTICE
Working with Difficult Emotions

The three approaches to difficult emotions described above can be practiced separately or together and are best applied in daily life, when you need them the most. You can use the following instructions to practice these skills or listen to a recording available online (see the end of the Contents for information).

- Find a comfortable position, sitting or lying down, close your eyes, and take three relaxing breaths.

- Place your hand on your heart, or another soothing place, for a few moments to remind yourself that you are in the room, and that you, too, are worthy of kindness.

- Let yourself recall a *mild to moderately difficult situation* that you are in right now, perhaps a health problem, stress in a relationship, or a loved one in pain. Do not choose a very difficult problem or a trivial problem—choose a problem that can generate a little stress in your body when you think of it.

- Clearly visualize the situation. *Who is involved? What's happening?*

Labeling Emotions

- As you relive this situation, notice if any emotions arise within you. And if so, see if a *label* for an emotion comes up, a *name*. For example:
    - Anger
    - Sadness
    - Grief
    - Confusion
    - Fear
    - Longing
    - Despair

- If you are having many emotions, see if you have a name for the *strongest* emotion associated with the situation.

- Now repeat the name of the emotion to yourself in a gentle, understanding voice, as if you were validating for a friend what she was feeling: "That's longing." "That's grief."

Awareness of Emotions in the Body

- Now expand your awareness to your body as a whole.

- Recall the difficult situation again and scan your body for where you feel it most easily. In your mind's eye, sweep your body from head to toe, stopping where you can sense a little tension or discomfort.

- Just feel what is "feelable" in your body right now. Nothing more.

- Now if you can, *choose a single location in your body* where the feeling expresses itself most strongly, perhaps as a point of muscle tension, a hollow feeling, or even a heartache.

- In your mind, incline gently toward that spot. Allow your awareness to fully inhabit the physical sensation of the emotion in your body.

Soften–Soothe–Allow

- Now **soften** into the location in your body where you feel the difficult emotion. Let the muscles soften, let them relax, as if in warm water. Soften . . . soften . . . soften . . . Remember that we're not trying to change the feeling—we're just holding it in a tender way.

- If you wish, just soften a little around the edges.

- Now **soothe** yourself because of this difficult situation.

- If you wish, place your hand over the part of your body that feels uncomfortable and just feel the gentle touch of your hand. Perhaps imagining warmth and kindness flowing through your hand into your body. Maybe even thinking of your body as if it were the body of a beloved child.

- And are there some comforting words that you might need to hear? If so, imagine you had a friend who was struggling in the same way. What would you say to your friend? ("I'm so sorry you feel this way." "I care deeply about you.") Can you offer yourself a similar message? ("Oh, it's so hard to feel this." "May I be kind to myself.")

- If you need to, feel free to open your eyes whenever you wish or let go of the exercise and just feel your breath.

- Finally, *allow* the discomfort to be there. Make room for it, releasing the need to make it go away.

- Allow *yourself* to be just as you are, just like this, if only for this moment.

- If you wish, you can repeat the cycle with your emotion, going a bit deeper each time, sticking with the sensation if it moves in your body or even morphs into a different emotion. Soften . . . soothe . . . allow. Soften . . . soothe . . . allow.

- Now let go of the practice and focus on your body as a whole. Allow yourself to feel whatever you feel, to be exactly as you are in this moment.

REFLECTION

Did you notice a change when you *labeled* the emotion? What did you observe when you *explored your body* for the physical sensation associated with the emotion? What happened when you *softened* that part of the body, *soothed* yourself, and *allowed* it to be there? Did the emotion change during the exercise, or did the physical manifestation move around your body a little? Did you encounter any difficulties with this practice?

Some people have difficulty finding a location in their body that corresponds to an emotion. One reason is that some people just have more awareness of body sensation than others (a skill called "interoception"). Another reason is that we may go numb when an emotion is too strong. In any case, you can focus on whatever is there, perhaps a more general sense of uneasiness in the body, or even numbness, with compassionate awareness.

Sometimes the emotion that first appears changes into a different emotion, or changes location. For instance, what may start out as the emotion of fear and tension behind the eyes could morph into grief residing in the pit of one's stomach. As we are able to identify, feel, and compassionately allow ourselves to experience our emotions, we often uncover deeper layers of emotion lying underneath.

If you start feeling overwhelmed as you do any practices in this book, let the exercise go until you feel safe and comfortable again. Healing takes time, and our limits must be respected. Walk slowly, go farther.

17

Self-Compassion and Shame

Shame stems from the innocent desire to be loved—to be worthy of affection and to belong. We are all born with the wish to be loved. When we manage to be loved as infants, everything we need comes our way—food, clothing, shelter, and connection. As adults, we still need each other to survive—to raise children and to protect ourselves from danger. Shame is the feeling that something is fundamentally wrong with us that will render us unacceptable or unlovable. One of the reasons shame is so intense is that it feels like our very survival is at stake.

Shame actually has three curious paradoxes:

- Shame feels blameworthy, but it is an innocent emotion.
- Shame feels lonely and isolating, but it is a universal emotion.
- Shame feels permanent and all-encompassing, but it is a transitory emotional state that only corresponds to part of who we are.

Arun was an upper-level manager at a health insurance company but would become paralyzed by feelings of shame whenever he had to speak in front of a group at work. No matter how prepared or knowledgeable he was about the topic, Arun felt inarticulate and bumbling and was certain other people would figure out he was an imposter who shouldn't be in a position of authority. Arun wanted so badly to be considered a good leader but was constantly fighting feelings of inadequacy. It didn't help that English was his second language. After one of these "shame attacks," as he called them, Arun would often lock the door of his office and hide.

There is a difference between guilt and shame. Guilt refers to feeling bad about a behavior; shame is feeling bad about ourselves. Guilt says I *did* something bad;

shame says I *am* bad. Guilt can actually be a productive emotion because it motivates us to repair situations when needed. Shame is typically unproductive, however, because it paralyzes us and renders us incapable of effective action. Research shows that self-compassion allows us to experience our feelings of sadness, regret, and guilt without getting trapped by feelings of shame.

> *Guilt is about our behavior; shame is about ourselves.*

Negative Core Beliefs

There are specific, repetitive thoughts that go through our minds when life becomes difficult—lingering self-doubts, often originating in childhood, that seem patently clear and true in our most vulnerable moments. These are our negative core beliefs that lie at the root of shame. Some examples are:

- "I'm defective."
- "I'm unlovable."
- "I'm helpless."
- "I'm inadequate."
- "I'm a failure."

Actually, the common negative core beliefs that human beings have about themselves are limited in number, perhaps as few as 15–20. Since there are over 7 billion people on the planet, we can conclude that whatever imperfection we think separates us from the rest of humanity may actually be shared by half a billion people!

Shame is maintained by silence. Negative core beliefs persist because we hide them from others (and from ourselves). We fear that we will be rejected if these aspects of ourselves were known. We forget that other people have the same feelings we do and also feel abnormal and isolated. When we reveal our negative core beliefs, at least to ourselves, they begin to lose their power over us.

> *Hiding our shame keeps it alive.*

We all have strengths and weaknesses. We can't sum ourselves up as simply worthy or unworthy, lovable or unlovable. As human beings, we're too multifaceted and complex. Self-compassion embraces all parts of ourselves in warm, openhearted awareness. When we are convinced that we are fatally flawed, have always been this way, and always will be, it really means that we are absorbed in one part and can't see the rest of ourselves. We need to embrace this part, with its negative core belief, and acknowledge our whole self, to be set free.

After years of struggling with his "shame attacks," Arun had finally had enough. He wasn't going to let feelings of inadequacy spoil his success. He knew that his shame had its roots in the fact that his father always favored his older brother, Dev, praising him for his achievements while pointing out all the ways Arun-ji (his nickname) needed to improve. So Arun began to form a new relationship with his child-self, the part of him who felt he could never measure up. When feelings of shame or inadequacy arose, Arun would imagine putting his arm around little Arun-ji, saying kind, encouraging things to him. "You're going to do great, and if you make a mistake, that's okay too. I'll accept and be here for you no matter what." Arun also set a photo of himself at that age on his desk at home and talked to it in the way he wished his father had spoken to him.

After several months of this practice, Arun started to be more confident speaking at company meetings. His shame didn't go away, but he wasn't disabled by it anymore, and in fact Arun learned to become friends with this part of himself. After all, Arun was a grown man with a great deal of knowledge and experience. This wiser and more mature part of Arun knew very well how to provide the support that little Arun-ji needed.

Self-compassion is the ultimate antidote to shame. By relating to our mistakes with kindness rather than self-judgment, remembering our common humanity instead of feeling isolated by our failures, and being mindful of our negative emotions (I feel bad) rather than identifying with them (I am bad), self-compassion directly dismantles the edifice of shame. And by holding our entire experience—including the experience of shame—in loving, connected presence, we become whole again.

 EXERCISE

Working with Our Negative Core Beliefs

Our negative core beliefs about ourselves are just that—beliefs and not reality. They are thoughts that are deeply ingrained in our psyche, often formed in our youth, which typically hold very little truth value. When these thoughts remain unconscious, however, they have a lot of power over us. An important first step is identifying and becoming aware of these thoughts. When we hold these beliefs up to the light of day, their power starts to dissolve. It's like lifting the curtain on the Wizard of Oz, revealing that he is not the great and mighty ruler he claims to be, but an ordinary con man from Kansas.

Still, it can be challenging to work with negative core beliefs, especially for those people who have experienced childhood trauma. Check in with yourself to determine if you are in the right mental and emotional space to do this exercise—perhaps the more self-compassionate thing to do would be to take a pass. Or if you are currently seeing a therapist, it may make more sense to do this exercise with some guidance and support from a professional.

Instructions

Here is a list of common negative core beliefs. Note any beliefs you may sometimes hold and try to identify if there is a particular context in which they arise (at work, in relationships, with your family, etc.).

I am not good enough	I am defective	I am a failure
I am stupid	I am helpless	I am incapable
I am a fraud	I am bad	I am unlovable
I am unwanted	I am worthless	I am unimportant
I am abnormal	I am weak	I am powerless

Next, see if you can bring the three components of self-compassion to bear on your negative core beliefs.

- *Mindfulness*: Write in an objective and validating manner about what it feels like to hold these negative beliefs. For example, "It's so painful when I have the thought that I am unlovable" or "It's very hard to feel that I am powerless."

- *Common humanity*: Write about how your beliefs are part of human experience. For example, "There are probably millions of people who feel like I do" or "I am not alone in feeling this way."

- *Kindness.* Now write some words of understanding and kindness to yourself, expressing concern for the suffering you've experienced because of this negative core belief. You might try writing to yourself as if you were speaking to a friend who just admitted she had this belief about herself. For example, "I'm so sorry you feel this way. I can see how painful it is for you. Please know that I don't believe this about you."

REFLECTION

What was this exercise like for you? Were you able to identity one or two negative core beliefs? How did it feel to bring mindfulness, common humanity, and kindness to the experience of having this belief?

Sometimes people find that when they try to hold their negative core beliefs in compassion the beliefs just assert themselves even more strongly. It may be that backdraft is occurring (see Chapter 8)—the love is rushing in and the old pain is rushing out. Another common occurrence is that the part of ourselves that has identified with the negative core belief feels frightened, as if we are trying to do away with this part. It's important to remember that we aren't trying to get rid of our negative core beliefs or make them go away. Rather, we are simply trying to relate to them in a more conscious, caring way so they don't have such power over us.

INFORMAL PRACTICE
Working with Shame

This practice is similar to Working with Difficult Emotions (see Chapter 16). We can label the cognitive component of shame—the negative core belief—as well as where shame resides in the body, and then bring compassion to the experience. Of particular importance when dismantling shame is remembering it comes from the wish to be loved, it's nearly universal, and it's an emotion, so therefore transitory. These elements are woven through the following practice.

Once again, make sure you do this practice only if you feel it is the right thing for you at this time. If you do decide to do the practice and become uncomfortable at any time, please take care of yourself and stop if needed. For example, you can take a warm bath or pet your dog, or just take a walk, feeling the soles of your feet (see Chapter 8).

In the following practice, you will be encouraged to focus more on embarrassment than shame. We are building resources and want to proceed slowly.

- Find a comfortable position, sitting or lying down, and close your eyes, partially or fully, and take few deep, relaxing breaths. You can even give a little sigh if you want. *Ahhhhhhhhh.*

- Place your hand over your heart or another soothing place, reminding yourself that you are in the room, perhaps allowing kindness to flow through your hand into your body.

- Now bring to mind an event that made you feel *embarrassed* or *somewhat ashamed.* For example:
  - You may have overreacted to something.
  - You may have said something stupid.
  - You may have blown a work assignment.
  - You may have realized your zipper was open at an important social event.

- Choose an event that is disturbing enough that you can feel it in your body. If it doesn't make you feel uneasy, choose another, but make it about a 3 on a scale from 1 to 10.

- Let it be an event that *you would not like anyone to hear about,* or remember, because it would probably make someone else think less of you.

- For now, choose a situation that makes you feel bad about yourself, not one that hurt others and may make you feel the need to ask someone for forgiveness.

- Feel your way into it, remembering the event in some detail. This takes some courage. Use all your senses, especially noting how shame or embarrassment feels in your body.

Labeling Core Beliefs

- Now, reflect for a moment and see if you can determine precisely *what it is that you're afraid others might discover about you.* Can you give it a name? Perhaps "I'm defective," "I'm unkind," "I'm a fraud." These are negative core beliefs.

- If you found a few of them, choose the one that seems to carry the most weight.

- As you go into this, you may already be feeling alone. If you are feeling this way, recognize that we are "alone together"—everyone feels exactly as you are feeling at one point or another. Shame is a universal emotion.

- Now name the core belief for yourself in a way that you might name it for a friend. For example, "Oh, you've been thinking that you are unlovable. That must be so painful!" Or just say to yourself in a warm, compassionate voice, "Unlovable. I think I'm unlovable!"

- Remember that when we feel embarrassed or ashamed, it is only *part* of us that feels this way. We don't always feel like this, although the feeling may seem very old and familiar.

- And our negative core beliefs arise out of the *wish to be loved.* We are all innocent beings, wishing to be loved.

- As a reminder, please know that you can open your eyes anytime during this exercise if it becomes uncomfortable, or otherwise disengage in any way you like.

Mindfulness of Shame in the Body

- Now expand your awareness to your body as a whole.

- Recall the difficult situation again and scan your body for where you feel embarrassment or shame most readily. In your mind's eye, sweep your body from head to toe, stopping where you can sense a little tension or discomfort.

- Now *choose a single location in your body* where shame or embarrassment expresses itself most strongly, perhaps as a point of muscle tension, hollowness, or a heartache. You don't need to be too specific.

- Again, please take good care of yourself as you go through this exercise.

Soften–Soothe–Allow

- Now, in your mind, gently incline toward that location in your body.

- *Soften* into that area. Let the muscles soften, letting them relax, as if in warm water. Soften . . . soften . . . soften. . . . Remember that we're not trying to change the feeling—we're just holding it in a tender way. If you wish, just soften a little around the edges.

- Now *soothe* yourself because of this difficult situation. If you wish, place your hand over the part of your body that holds embarrassment or shame and just feel the warmth and gentle touch of your hand, acknowledging how hard that part of our body has been working to hold this emotion. If you like, imagine warmth and kindness flowing through your hand into your body. Maybe even think of your body as if it were the body of a beloved child.

- And are there some comforting words that you might need to hear? If so, imagine you had a friend who was struggling in the same way. What would you say to your friend, heart to heart? ("I'm so sorry you feel this way." "I care deeply about you.") What do you want your friend to know, to remember?

- Now, try offering yourself the same message. ("Oh, it's so hard to feel this." "May I be kind to myself.") Let the words in, to whatever extent possible.

- Again, remember that when we feel embarrassed or ashamed, that it is only part of us that feels that way. We don't always feel like this.

- Finally, *allow* the discomfort to be there, letting your body have whatever sensations it is having and your heart to feel as it does. Make room for everything and release the need to make anything go away.

- If you wish, you can repeat the cycle, going a bit deeper each time. Soften . . . soothe . . . allow. Soften . . . soothe . . . allow.

- Before we close the practice, just remember that you are connected right now to everyone in the world who has ever experienced embarrassment or shame and that it comes from the wish to be loved.

- Now let go of the practice and focus on your body as a whole. Allow yourself to feel whatever you feel, to be exactly as you are in this moment.

REFLECTION

Were you able to identify a negative core belief behind the experience of embarrassment or shame? How did it feel to name the core belief?

Could you find shame in your body? If so, where?

Did softening, soothing, or allowing shift the experience of shame in any way?

It can be very challenging to work with shame. It probably took some courage to get as far as you did, but if you didn't complete the exercise because you were practicing self-care, thank yourself for that as well.

A variety of obstacles may arise as you do this practice. For example, it might be difficult to feel shame in the body. Shame can be a precursor to spacing out, and sometimes shame is felt as emptiness or a void in the body, particularly in the head. You can actually focus on the feeling of nothingness, though it is difficult to do so. People also find it challenging to give themselves compassion when they're in the grip of shame because they feel undeserving. And it's highly likely that our familiar friend backdraft arose for you during this practice (see Chapter 8). If this exercise was difficult for you for any reason, just shift your focus to a tender appreciation of the struggle. That's practicing self-compassion.

18

Self-Compassion in Relationships

Much of our suffering arises in relationship with others. As Sartre famously wrote, "Hell is other people." The good news is that much of our relationship suffering is unnecessary and can be prevented by cultivating a loving relationship with ourselves.

There are at least two types of relational pain. One is the pain of *connection*—when those we care about are suffering (see Chapter 19).

The other type is the pain of *disconnection*—when we experience loss or rejection and feel hurt, angry, or alone (see Chapter 20).

Our capacity for emotional resonance means that emotions are contagious. This is especially true in intimate relationships. If you are irritated with your partner but try to hide it, for instance, your partner will often pick up on your irritation. He might say, "Are you angry at me?" Even if you deny it, your partner will feel the irritation; it will affect his mood, leading to an irritated tone of voice. You will feel this, in turn, and become even more irritated, and your responses will have a harsher tone, and on it goes. This is because our brains would have been communicating emotions to one another regardless of how carefully we chose our words.

> A downward spiral of negative emotions in an interaction can be replaced by an upward spiral when self-compassion is brought into play.

In social interactions, there can be a *downward spiral* of negative emotions—when one person has a negative attitude, the other person becomes even more negative, and so on. This means that other people are partly responsible for our state of mind, but we are also partly responsible for *their* state of mind. The good news is that emotional contagion gives us more power than we realize to change the emotional tenor of our relationships. Self-compassion can interrupt a downward spiral and start an upward spiral instead.

Compassion is actually a positive emotion and activates the reward centers of our brain, even though it arises in the presence of suffering. A very useful way to change the direction of a negative relationship interaction, therefore, is to have compassion for the pain we're feeling in the moment. The positive feelings of compassion we have for ourselves will also be felt by others—manifested in our tone and subtle facial expressions—and help to interrupt the negative cycle. In this way cultivating self-compassion is one of the best things we can do for our relationship interactions as well as for ourselves.

Not surprisingly, research shows that self-compassionate people have happier and more satisfying romantic relationships. In one study, for instance, individuals with higher levels of self-compassion were described by their partners as being more accepting and nonjudgmental than those who lacked self-compassion. Rather than trying to change their partners, self-compassionate people tended to respect their opinions and consider their point of view. They were also described as being more caring, connected, affectionate, intimate, and willing to talk over relationship problems than those who lacked self-compassion. At the same time, self-compassionate people were described as giving their partners more freedom and autonomy in their relationships. They tended to encourage partners to make their own decisions and to follow their own interests. In contrast, people who lacked self-compassion were described as being more critical and controlling of their partners. They were also described as being more self-centered, inflexibly wanting everything their own way.

Steve met Sheila in college, and after 15 years of marriage he still loved her dearly. He hated to admit this to himself, but she was also starting to drive him crazy. Sheila was terribly insecure and constantly needed Steve to reassure her of his love and affection. Wasn't sticking around for 15 years enough? If he didn't tell her "I love you" every day, she would start to worry, and if a few days went by she got into a proper sulk. He felt controlled by her need for reassurance and resented the fact that she didn't honor his own need to express himself authentically. Their relationship was starting to suffer.

To have the type of close, connected relationships we really want with others, we first need to feel close and connected to *ourselves*. By being supportive toward ourselves in times of struggle, we gain the emotional resources needed to care for our significant others. When we meet our own needs for love and acceptance, we can place fewer demands on our partners, allowing them to be more fully themselves. Cultivating self-compassion is far from selfish. It gives us the resilience we need to build and sustain happy and healthy relationships in our lives.

> *Close connections with others start with feeling connected to ourselves.*

Over time Sheila was able to see how her constant need for reassurance from Steve was driving him away. She realized that she had become a black hole and that Steve would never be able to fully satisfy her insecurity by giving her "enough" love. It would never be enough. So Sheila started a practice of journaling at night to give herself the love and affection she craved. She would write the type of tender words to herself that she was hoping to hear from Steve, like "I love you sweetheart. I won't ever leave you." Then, first thing in the morning, she would read what she had written and let it soak in. She began giving herself the reassurance she was desperately seeking from Steve and let him off the hook. It wasn't quite as nice, she had to admit, but she liked the fact that she wasn't so dependent. As the pressure eased, Steve started to be more naturally expressive in their relationship, and they became closer. The more secure she felt in her own self-acceptance, the more she was able to accept his love as it was, not just how she wanted it to be. Ironically, by meeting her own needs she became less self-focused and started to feel an independence that was new and delicious.

INFORMAL PRACTICE

Self-Compassion Break in Relationship Conflicts

- The next time you're in a negative interaction with someone, try using the Self-Compassion Break (Chapter 4). You can excuse yourself for a moment, or if you can't leave, practice the Self-Compassion Break silently: "This is a moment of suffering." "Suffering is part of any relationship." "May I be kind to myself." It helps to use some sort of supportive touch. If you're alone, you can put a hand on your heart or elsewhere, but if you're in the presence of someone else, you may want to practice a more subtle form of touch, such as holding your own hand.

- Before reengaging with the other person, try practicing Giving and Receiving Compassion (Chapter 15) to maintain your caring attitude. Breathe in for yourself, acknowledging the pain you are feeling in the moment, then breathe out for the other. Make sure you fully validate your own pain and give yourself what you need as well as honoring the struggle of the other person.

- Notice how the state of mind of the other person may change as your own state of mind changes.

REFLECTION

After trying out the Self-Compassion Break in your relationships a few times, do you notice any impact on your interactions?

It can be especially powerful if the other person in the relationship is aware of the idea of self-compassion and is also committed to practicing it. In this case, especially if an interaction is becoming heated, just one of you has to remember to call out "Self-compassion break!" and then you can both take a pause, give yourself compassion for any pain that is arising, and start again.

EXERCISE

Fulfilling Our Emotional Needs

We often put pressure on our relationships when we expect our partners to magically intuit and then meet all of our emotional needs. For example, if you resent the fact that your partner didn't realize you needed encouragement and a hug to get one project done, but that on another project what you actually needed was more space and time to yourself, your partner will suffer under the weight of superhuman expectations. You will also suffer because your needs aren't being met. Instead of relying on your partner to give you exactly what you need, you can try meeting your own needs directly. Of course we can't meet all of our own needs and must still rely on other people, but we aren't as wholly dependent as we might think.

- Take out a sheet of paper and write down any ways that you may be feeling dissatisfied in your relationship. For instance, maybe you feel you aren't getting enough attention from your partner, or respect, support, or validation? Instead of focusing on specifics (e.g., I don't get as many text messages as I would like), see if you can identify the particular need that isn't being met—to be valued, cared for, and so forth.

- Now write down some ideas for how you might try to meet your need yourself. For instance, if you would like a sign of being cared for, can you buy yourself flowers? If you need more touch, can you get a weekly massage or hold your own hand? Can you let yourself know you are loved and supported by using kind language with yourself? It may seem silly at first, but if we get in the habit of meeting some of our own needs, we will be less dependent on our partners for emotional fulfilment, and we will have more resources available to give.

REFLECTION

Many people find it a revelation that they can meet some of their own emotional needs for themselves rather than relying entirely on someone else to do it for them. Some also feel sadness, grief, or anger, however, at the fact that their partner isn't meeting their needs satisfactorily. Remember that meeting your own needs doesn't mean that your partner shouldn't *also* meet your needs, especially when you have communicated them clearly. A healthy relationship means both parties give and receive. However, this back-and-forth flow can usually occur more easily when both people are emotionally fulfilled by giving themselves kindness, support, and care.

 MEDITATION
Compassionate Friend

This visualization meditation will help you connect with the part of yourself that is compassionate by discovering an image for your compassionate self and starting a conversation with that image. Strengthening the relationship with your compassionate self is an important resource for strengthening your relationships with others. This meditation, adapted from the work of Paul Gilbert, is particularly helpful for people who have trouble developing self-compassion.

Some people are good visualizers, and others are not. Practice in a relaxed manner, allowing the meditation to unfold by itself and letting images come and go. If no images arise, that is also fine, and you can simply linger with the feelings that are present. (To find a guided recording of this meditation online, see the end of the Contents.)

- Find a comfortable position, either sitting or lying down. Gently close your eyes. Take a few deep breaths to settle into your body. Put one or two hands over your heart or another soothing place to remind yourself to give yourself *loving* attention.

Safe Place

- Imagine yourself in a place that is safe and comfortable—it might be a cozy room with the fireplace burning or a peaceful beach with warm sun and a cool breeze, or a forest glade. It could also be an imaginary place, like floating on clouds . . . anywhere you feel peaceful and safe. Let yourself linger with and enjoy the feeling of comfort in this place.

Compassionate Friend

- Soon you'll receive a visitor, a warm and caring presence—a compassionate friend—an imaginary figure who embodies the qualities of wisdom, strength, and unconditional love.

- This being may be a spiritual figure or a wise, compassionate teacher; she may embody qualities of someone you have known in the past, like a loving grandparent, or be completely from your imagination. This being may not have any particular form, perhaps just a presence or glowing light.

- Your compassionate friend cares deeply about you and would like you to be happy and free from unnecessary struggle.

- Allow an image to come to mind.

Arrival

- You have a choice to go out from your safe place and meet your compassionate friend or to invite him in. Take that opportunity now, if you like.

- Position yourself in just the right way in relation to your compassionate friend—whatever feels right. Then allow yourself to feel what it's like to be in the company of this being. There is nothing you need to do except to experience the moment.

- See if you can allow yourself to fully receive the unconditional love and compassion this being has for you, to soak it in. If you can't let it fully in, that's okay too—this being feels it anyway.

Meeting

- Your compassionate friend is wise and all-knowing and understands exactly where you are in your own life journey. Your friend might want to tell you something, something that is *just what you need to hear right now.* Take a moment and listen carefully to what your compassionate friend has come to say.

If no words come, that's okay, too—just experience the good company. That's a blessing in itself.

- And perhaps *you* would like to say something to your compassionate friend. Your friend will listen deeply and completely understands you. Is there anything *you'd* like to share?

- Your friend may also like to leave you with a gift—a material object. The object will simply appear in your hands, or you can put out your hands and receive one—something that has special meaning to you.

  If something appears, what is it?

- Now take a few more moments to enjoy your friend's presence. And as you continue to enjoy this being's good company, allow yourself to realize that your friend is actually part of yourself. All the compassionate feelings, images, and words that you experienced flow from your own inner wisdom and compassion.

Return

- Finally, when you're ready, allow the images to gradually dissolve in your mind's eye, remembering that compassion and wisdom are always within you, especially when you need them the most. You can call on your compassionate friend anytime you wish.

- Now settle back into your body, letting yourself savor what just happened, perhaps reflecting on the words you may have heard or the object that may have been given to you.

- And finally, let go of the meditation and allow yourself to feel whatever you feel and to be exactly as you are.

- Gently open your eyes.

REFLECTION

Could you visualize a safe place and feel the comfort of it? Did an image of a compassionate friend or a presence come to mind?

Did you hear something meaningful from your compassionate friend that spoke to what you need right now? What was it like to be able to speak to this being? Did you receive anything with special meaning?

Was this meditation challenging to you in any way? What was it like to discover that your compassionate friend is actually a part of yourself and that this being's compassion and wisdom are always available to you?

For visually oriented people, this meditation can be very powerful, especially as a way to hear the inner voice of compassion and address practical day-to-day concerns.

Sometimes the compassionate friend is someone who has passed away, such as a parent or grandparent, and feelings of grief may arise. If grief gets in the way of feeling the person's compassion, it may be helpful to switch to an entirely imaginary being who embodies the same qualities or a less clearly defined compassionate presence. If the grief isn't overwhelming, however, it can be a great treasure to discover that our loved one who has passed continues to live within us in the form of inner wisdom and compassion.

19

Self-Compassion for Caregivers

By the time most people reach midlife, they are caregivers in one form or another. Some might be caregivers in their professional careers—doctors, nurses, therapists, social workers, teachers—and others in their personal lives, caring for children, elderly parents, spouses, friends, and so on.

When we care for others who are suffering, the process of empathic resonance means that we feel their distress as our own (see Chapter 15). When we witness someone else in pain, the pain centers of our own brains become active. Empathic distress can be hard to bear, so it's natural to try to block it out or make it go away as we would any other pain, but the constant struggle can be draining and lead to caregiver fatigue and burnout.

How do we know we've reached the point of burnout? Usually there are signs such as being distracted, angry or irritated, restless, or avoidant of others, having trouble sleeping, or experiencing distressing and intrusive thoughts. Caregiver fatigue is not a sign of weakness, but a sign of caring. In fact, the more caregivers are capable of empathic resonance (which is what often draws people into caregiving professions), the more vulnerable they may be to caregiver fatigue. Human beings are limited in how much vicarious suffering they can take on without becoming overwhelmed.

Typically, there are two main types of advice given to prevent caregiver burnout. One is to draw clear emotional *boundaries* between ourselves and those we care for. The problem with this approach is that if you are a professional caregiver, emotional sensitivity is necessary to do an effective job, and if you are caring for a loved one like a child or a parent, the drawing of boundaries can harm the quality of the relationship.

The other type of advice given to prevent burnout is to engage in *self-care* activities. These are typically behaviors like exercising, eating well, spending time with friends, or going on vacation. While self-care is extremely important, there is a big limitation to self-care strategies as a way to deal with caregiving burnout. Self-care tends to happen *off* the job and doesn't help us in the midst of caregiving interactions themselves. For example, we can't tell a therapy client who has just dropped a bombshell of a story, "Whoa, man, that story is freaking me out. I think I'll go get a massage!"

What role might compassion have here? Many people feel it is compassion that drains caregivers. That's why the phenomenon is often called "compassion fatigue." Some researchers argue that this is a misnomer, however, and that compassion fatigue is really "empathy fatigue."

> *Self-care is a limited antidote to caregiver burnout because it doesn't help us while we're giving care.*

What is the difference between empathy and compassion? Carl Rogers defined *empathy* as "an accurate understanding of the [client's] world as seen from the inside. To sense the client's private world as if it were your own." If we just resonate with the suffering of others without having the emotional resources to hold it, we will become exhausted. Compassion entails a sense of tenderness and care that embraces the suffering of others rather than struggling with it. Empathy says, "I *feel* you." Compassion says, "I *hold* you." Compassion is a positive emotion, an energizing emotion. One research study trained people for several days to experience empathy or compassion and then showed them a short film depicting others' suffering.

> *Where empathy says, "I feel you," compassion says, "I hold you" and produces positive emotions.*

The films activated distinctly different brain networks, and only compassion training activated networks associated with positive emotions.

It is crucial that we *give ourselves compassion* when experiencing empathic pain, as well as giving compassion to those we care for. As we are told whenever we fly, when there is a drop in cabin pressure, we need to put on our own oxygen mask first, before we help others. Some caregivers may believe they should *only* be concerned with the needs of others and are often self-critical because they think they aren't giving enough. However, if you don't meet your own emotional needs by giving yourself compassion, you will become depleted and less able to give.

Importantly, when you calm and soothe your own mind, the person you're caring for will also feel calmed and soothed through her own empathetic resonance. In other words, when we cultivate peace within, we help all those we're in contact with to become more peaceful as well.

We learned about the importance of self-compassion for caregivers firsthand. It helped us to thrive in our roles as caregivers—one as the parent of a child with autism and the other as a therapist—without burning out.

I (Kristin) was on a transatlantic flight with my son, Rowan. For some reason, just at the moment when they dimmed the lights in the cabin and the passengers hoped to get some sleep, Rowan lost it. A full-on screaming, flailing tantrum. He was about five years old at the time. I remember feeling like every person on the plane was looking at us: What's wrong with that kid? He's too old to be acting like this. What's wrong with that mother? Why can't she control her child? At a loss for what to do, I thought I would take Rowan to the toilet and let him scream there, and hopefully his cries would be muffled. No luck. Occupied.

So as I sat with Rowan outside the toilet in the little cubicle of space we had, I knew I had no choice but to give myself compassion. I breathed in compassion for myself, put my hand on my heart, and silently supported myself. "This is so hard for you, darling. I'm so sorry this is happening. It will be okay. It will pass." I made sure Rowan was safe, but 95% of my attention was focused on soothing and comforting myself. Then I observed something that I often observed with Rowan. As I calmed down, he calmed down. I had learned that in those moments when I forgot my self-compassion practice and became agitated, Rowan would get more agitated, but when I gave myself compassion for the pain of the situation, Rowan would become more peaceful. He was resonating with my emotions just as much as I was resonating with his. By tending to my own feelings of overwhelm first, moreover, I gained the stability needed to fully be there for Rowan, and to love and support him unconditionally despite the difficulty. I quickly learned that practicing self-compassion—entering a state of loving, connected presence in the midst of suffering—was one of the most effective ways I could help Rowan as well as myself.

I (Chris) had agreed to see a patient for therapy even though I didn't have much time in my schedule. When the patient, Franco, came through the door, he looked much more depressed than he had sounded on the phone. His shoulders were hunched and his face looked drawn. Soon into our session, Franco told me that he had lined up all his medications by his bedside and that he was comforted by the thought that he could end his life at any time. His wife had recently left him, he was marginally employed, and that morning he had received an eviction notice from his landlord.

When Franco arrived, I felt nothing but curiosity and compassion for this new person. However, when he mentioned suicide, I felt fear coursing through my body and regretted that I had ever agreed to see Franco. Learning about the difficult situation Franco was in only increased my fear that Franco would try to harm himself.

Knowing that a genuine emotional connection is often what keeps a person alive through a dark night of the soul, I realized I needed to try to stay connected with Franco despite my fear. I took a long inbreath for myself, reminding myself that this is part of the job of a psychologist, and slowly exhaled for Franco. Again and again I did this until I could listen to Franco's story with an open heart and less fear. I also reminded myself that I could not be responsible for saving Franco's life, but I would do whatever I could do in my capacity as a therapist. Breathing in this way, and reminding myself of the limits of my ability to control the situation, gave me space to feel Franco's despair in my own body. When I shared with Franco how moved I felt by his situation, Franco softened and began to explain to me all the courageous steps he was taking to stay alive and get through the crisis. When Franco left my office, we both had a ray of hope.

EXERCISE
Reducing Stress for Caregivers

If you're a caregiver, it's important to make wise choices of activities to engage in so that you aren't overloaded. Although it's impossible to get rid of stress entirely, you can do a lot to help. In each of the life domains below, identify those helpful behaviors that you currently engage in that help you cope with the stress of being a caregiver, those unhelpful activities that *add* to your stress level, and then note any ideas for changes you might make to take better care of yourself as a caregiver.

Physical activities (e.g., diet, exercise, sleep)

Helpful? _____

Unhelpful? _____

Changes? _____

Psychological activities (e.g., therapy, books, music)

Helpful? _____

Unhelpful? _____

Changes? _____

Relationship activities (e.g., family, groups, intimacy)

Helpful? _____

Unhelpful? _____

Changes? _____

Work activities (e.g., hours per week, screen time, breaks)

Helpful? _____

Unhelpful? _____

Changes? _____

INFORMAL PRACTICE
Compassion with Equanimity

This practice combines Giving and Receiving Compassion with the practice of equanimity, or balance in the midst of difficulty. Adding equanimity is especially important in caregiving situations because it reminds us of our limited control over others' suffering and allows us to get more perspective so that compassion can arise. This practice can actually be applied to any challenging relationship interaction but is especially powerful for caregivers. (A

> *As a caregiver, can you also meet your own needs— soothe, comfort, protect, and provide for yourself?*

guided recording of this practice is available online; see the end of the Contents for information.)

- Find a comfortable position and take a few deep breaths to settle into your body and into the present moment. You might like to put your hand over your heart, or wherever it is comforting and soothing, as a reminder to bring affectionate awareness to your experience and to yourself.

- Bring to mind someone you are caring for who is exhausting you or frustrating you—someone you care about who is suffering. For this introductory exercise, choose someone who is *not* your child, as this can be a more complicated dynamic. Visualize the person and the caregiving situation clearly in your mind and feel the struggle in your own body.

- Now read these words, letting them gently roll through your mind:

We are each on our own life journey.
I am not the cause of this person's suffering,
nor is it entirely within my power to make it go away,
even though I wish I could.
Moments like this are difficult to bear,
yet I may still try to help if I can.

Aware of the stress you are carrying in your body, inhale fully and deeply, drawing compassion inside your body and filling every cell of your body with compassion. Let yourself be soothed by inhaling deeply and by giving yourself the compassion you need.

- As you exhale, send out compassion to the person who is associated with your discomfort.

- Continue breathing compassion in and out, allowing your body to gradually find a natural, breathing rhythm—letting your body breathe itself.

- "One for me, one for you." "In for me, out for you."

- Occasionally scan your inner landscape for any distress and respond by inhaling compassion for yourself and exhaling compassion for the other.

- If you find that anyone needs *extra* compassion, focus your attention and your breath more in that direction.

- Let yourself float on an ocean of compassion—a limitless, boundless ocean that embraces all suffering.

- And take in these words once again:

We are each on our own life journey.
I am not the cause of this person's suffering,
nor is it entirely within my power to make it go away,
even though I wish I could.
Moments like this are difficult to bear,
yet I may still try to help if I can.

- Now let go of the practice and allow yourself to be exactly as you are in this moment.
- Gently open your eyes.

REFLECTION

What did you notice or feel while doing this practice? Did you experience an internal shift when you said the equanimity phrases? Were you able to adjust the "flow" of compassion inward or outward, as needed?

Breathing "in for me and out for you" ensures that caregivers don't forget compassion for themselves. Together with equanimity, this practice is a deceptively simple way to stay connected and emotionally disentangled at the same time. The equanimity phrases come as a special relief to caregivers who may take on too much responsibility for the suffering of those they are caring for. Our capacity to help is limited by the fact that we have separate bodies and separate lives. We do the best we can. What is less limited, however, is our ability to experience compassion. Giving compassion to oneself takes nothing away from giving to others, and in fact merely increases our capacity.

Equanimity is trickier for parents, especially of young children, but parents eventually understand that even their own children have separate, unique lives and life trajectories. In one MSC class, a mother who was breastfeeding her infant said that when she was breathing in for herself, she felt nauseous, as if she were depriving her daughter of life itself. Shortly thereafter, another participant quipped, "Well, I'm the mother of four children who have all left home, and I breathed in one for me, and . . . well . . . one for all four of you!"

20

Self-Compassion and Anger in Relationships

Another type of relational pain is *disconnection,* which occurs whenever there is a loss or rupture in a relationship. Anger is a common reaction to disconnection. We might get angry when we feel rejected or dismissed, but also when disconnection is unavoidable, such as when someone dies. The reaction may not be rational, but it still happens. Anger has a way of popping up around disconnection and can sometimes linger for years, long after the relationship has ended.

Although anger gets a bad rap, it isn't necessarily bad. Like all emotions, anger has positive functions. For instance, anger can give us information that someone has overstepped our boundaries or hurt us in some way, and it may be a powerful signal that something needs to change. Anger can also provide us with the energy and determination to protect ourselves in the face of threat, take action to stop harmful behavior, or end a toxic relationship.

While anger in and of itself is not a problem, we often have an unhealthy relationship with anger. For instance, we may not allow ourselves to feel our anger and suppress it instead. (This can be especially true for women, who are taught to be "nice," i.e., not angry.) When we try to stuff down our anger, it can lead to anxiety, emotional constriction, or numbness. Sometimes we turn the anger against ourselves in the form of harsh self-criticism, which is a surefire way to become depressed. And if we get stuck in angry rumination—who did what to whom and what they

> *Anger can be a perfectly healthy emotional response, but our relationship with it is often unhealthy.*

144

deserve for it—we live with an agitated state of mind and may end up getting angry at others for no apparent reason.

> *Nate was an electrician who lived in Chicago. He had split from his wife, Lila, over five years ago, but he still got enraged every time he thought about her. It turns out that Lila had an affair with a close friend of theirs, someone they often socialized with, and that this went on behind his back for almost a year. As soon as Nate found out about it, he was seething with anger. He somehow managed to refrain from calling her every name in the book, but he was sick to his stomach whenever he thought about what had happened. He filed for divorce almost immediately—thank goodness they didn't have children—so the process was relatively quick and easy. Although he hadn't had any contact with Lila for several years, his anger never really subsided. And the trauma of the affair kept Nate from forming new relationships because he had such a hard time trusting anyone.*

If we continually harden our emotions in an attempt to protect ourselves against those we're angry at, over time we may develop *bitterness* and *resentment*. Anger, bitterness, and resentment are "hard feelings." Hard feelings are resistant to change and often stick with us long past the time when they are useful. (How many of us are still angry at someone we are unlikely to ever see again?) Furthermore, chronic anger causes chronic stress, which is bad for all the systems of the body—cardiovascular, endocrine, nervous, even the reproductive system. As the saying goes, "Anger corrodes the vessel that contains it." Or "Anger is the poison we drink to kill another person." When anger is no longer helpful to us, the most compassionate thing we can do is change our relationship to it, especially by applying the resources of mindfulness and self-compassion.

How? The first step is to identify the *soft feelings* behind the hard feelings of anger. Often anger is protecting more tender, sensitive emotions, such as feeling hurt, scared, unloved, alone, or vulnerable. When we peel back the outer layer of anger to see what is underneath, we are often surprised by the fullness and complexity of our feelings. Hard feelings are difficult to work with directly because they are typically defensive and outward focused. When we identify our soft feelings, however, we turn inward and can begin the transformation process.

To truly heal, however, we need to peel back the layers even further and discover the *unmet needs* that are giving rise to our soft feelings. Unmet needs are universal human needs—those experiences that are core to any human being. The Center for Nonviolent Communication offers a comprehensive list of needs at *www.cnvc.org/ training/needs-inventory*. Some examples are the need to be safe, connected, validated, heard, included, autonomous, and respected. And our deepest need as human beings is the need to be loved.

By having the courage to turn toward and experience our authentic feelings and needs, we can begin to have insight into what is really going on for us. Once we contact the pain and respond with self-compassion, things can start to transform on a deep level. We can use self-compassion to meet our needs directly.

As discussed in Chapter 18, self-compassion in response to unmet needs means that we can begin to give ourselves what we have yearned to receive from others, perhaps for many years. We can be our own source of support, respect, love, validation, or safety. Of course, we need relationships and connection with others. We aren't automatons. But when others are unable to meet our needs, for whatever reason, and have harmed us in the process, we can recover by holding the hurt, the soft feelings, in a compassionate embrace and fill the hole in our hearts with loving, connected presence.

Nate worked hard at transforming his anger because he realized it was holding him back. He had tried catharsis to get it out—punching pillows, yelling at the top of his lungs—but it didn't work. Eventually Nate signed up for an MSC course because a friend was very enthusiastic about it and said it would reduce his stress.

When Nate came to the part of the MSC course that focused on transforming anger by meeting his unmet needs, he felt nervous but did it anyway. It was easy to get in touch with his anger, and even the hurt behind it, and feel it in his body. The toughest part was identifying his unmet need. Certainly Nate felt betrayed and unloved, but that wasn't what seemed to be holding him back. Nate stuck with the exercise, and finally the unmet need revealed itself, and his whole body relaxed. Respect!

Nate came from a hardworking blue-collar family, and his parents were still happily married after 30 years. He tried to do everything right in his own marriage, to the best of his ability, and he took his vows very seriously. Honesty and respect were core values for Nate. Knowing that Lila would never give him the respect he needed—it was too late for that—he took the plunge and tried to give it to himself. "I respect you," he told himself. At first it felt silly and empty and hollow. So he paused and tried to say the words as if they were true. He thought about how much he had sacrificed to get his master electrician's certification and open a business, the long hours he had put in to pay the mortgage and build a savings account. "I respect you," he repeated, over and over, though it still just sounded like words. Then he thought of how honest and hardworking he had tried to be in his marriage, even though that wasn't enough for Lila. Very, very slowly, Nate started to take it in. Finally he put his hand on his heart and said it like he really meant it: "I respect you." He started to tear up, because he actually felt it. Once he did, the anger at his wife started to melt away. He began to see her unmet needs, different from his, for more closeness and affection. Not that what Lila did was okay, but Nate realized that her behavior had nothing to do with his worth or value as a person. He couldn't rely on any outside person—even one who was reliable and faithful—to give him the respect he needed. It had to come from within.

EXERCISE

Meeting Unmet Needs

The purpose of this informal practice is to bring mindfulness to old resentment and to respond to underlying unmet needs with self-compassion. This practice is designed to establish a new *relationship* to old hurts that made you angry, not to heal those wounds or those relationships. Therefore, let go of the need to feel better and just see what happens.

Choose a mild to moderately difficult relationship for this practice, not a traumatic relationship, as strong emotions may make it more difficult to complete the practice. Also, feel free to skip this practice right now if you feel emotionally vulnerable or disengage from it after you start if you become distressed.

- In the space provided, note a past relationship that you still feel bitter or angry about and then recall a *specific event* in that relationship that was mildly to moderately disturbing—a 3 on a bitterness scale of 1–10. Remember not to choose an experience that was traumatizing or that left lasting psychological scars.

- It's important for this exercise that you choose a relationship that is over—not ongoing—in which your anger *no longer serves a purpose* and *you're ready to let it go.* Take your time to find just the right relationship and event to work with.

- As you do this exercise, try to make a lot of room for whatever you experience, trying to be mindful of what happened without getting lost in the story line. Also, if at any point you feel you need to "close" or stop the exercise, please do so. Take care of yourself.

- Close your eyes for a moment and call to mind the relationship event.

Remember the details as vividly as possible, getting in touch with your anger and feeling it in your body.

- Know that it's completely natural for you to feel as you do, perhaps saying to yourself, "It's okay to feel angry—you were hurt! This is a natural human response to being hurt." Or "You are not alone. Lots of people would have felt this way."

- Allow yourself to *fully validate* the experience of being angry, while trying not to get too caught up in story lines of right or wrong.

- There is no need to move on from here if validating your anger is what you need the most right now. If that is the case, just skip the remaining instructions and remember that your anger is natural, and be kind to yourself for the pain you have been carrying, perhaps for many years.

Soft Feelings

- If it feels okay to move on, begin to peel back the anger and resentment—the hard feelings—and see what's underneath.

  Are there any soft feelings behind the hard feelings?

  ○ Hurt? Fear? Loneliness? Sadness? Grief?

- When you have identified a soft feeling, try naming it for yourself in a gentle, understanding voice, as if you were supporting a dear friend: "Oh, that's sadness" or "That's fear."

- Again, if you need to, you can stay right here. What feels right for you?

Unmet Needs

- If you feel ready to move on, see if you can release the person and the story line of this hurt, if only for a while. You may have thoughts of right and wrong. See if you can set those thoughts aside for a moment, asking yourself . . .

  "What basic human need do I have, or did I have at the time, that was not met?" The need to be . . .

  ○ Seen? Heard? Safe? Connected? Respected? Special? Loved?

- What was your need that didn't get met?

- Again, try naming the need in a gentle, understanding voice.

Responding with Compassion

- If you wish to move on, try putting your hand on your body in a soothing way and give yourself some warmth and kindness, not to make the feelings go away but just because these feelings are arising.

- The hands that have been reaching outward—longing to receive care and support from others—can become the hands that give you the care and support that you need.

- Even though you wished to have your needs met by another person, he was unable to do so for a variety of reasons. But we have another resource—ourselves—and we can consider meeting these needs more directly.

  ○ If you needed to be seen, try saying "I see you." "I care."
  ○ If you needed to feel connected, try saying "I'm here for you." "You belong."
  ○ If you needed to feel loved, try saying "I love you." "You matter to me."

In other words, can you try to give yourself right now what you may have been longing to receive from someone else, perhaps for a long, long time?

- See if you can *receive* these words. There may be disappointment that the other could not meet your needs, but is it possible that you can meet at least *some* of your needs for yourself, right now in this moment?

- And if you're having trouble doing so, can you also have compassion for that—for the pain we have as humans when our deepest needs are unmet?

- Now let go of the exercise and simply rest in your experience, letting this moment be exactly as it is and yourself exactly as you are.

REFLECTION

How did it feel to validate your anger? Could you find soft feelings behind the anger? Did you discover an unmet need? Could you experience some self-compassion for that unmet need and perhaps even meet the need directly?

Hopefully you went only as far into this practice as felt right to you. After connecting with feelings of anger over a past harm, some people just aren't ready to peel back the layers so that soft feelings and needs underneath are revealed. In that case, the most self-compassionate thing to do may be to just validate the anger itself and stop there. Others may be able to identify the soft feelings and unmet needs beneath their anger, but when they try to meet their own needs directly, a little voice says, "But I don't *want* to meet my own needs. I want [this person] to do it!" This usually means that there are feelings of hurt that have not been validated. Or it may simply be that the natural wish for an apology is asserting itself. Until that blessed day, however, consider the possibility of giving yourself what you have urgently needed, perhaps for quite some time.

EXERCISE
Fierce Compassion

When anger is used in the service of alleviating the suffering of oneself or others, or standing up for what's right, it can be called "fierce compassion." Some of our greatest historical figures, such as the Rev. Dr. Martin Luther King Jr., harnessed anger at injustice to catalyze social reform while keeping the flame of universal respect and compassion alive. In other words, compassion doesn't make us weak or passive or cause us to lose the ability to discern right from wrong. Compassion helps us to clearly see what's going on and to understand the complex reasons people act as they do. This allows us to take appropriate action to stop harmful behavior without sorting people into categories of "good" and "bad." In this way, fierce compassion, as opposed to reactive anger, helps us stand up to injustice without making a bad situation worse through blame or hatred.

- Take two or three deep breaths and close your eyes for a few moments to settle and center yourself. Try putting your hands over your heart or use some other soothing touch as a gesture of support and self-kindness.

- Think of a particular *social or political* situation that you strongly disagree with. Instead of just being angry about it, imagine how you would think and feel about it with a mindset of fierce compassion. Can you describe the situation in a way that does not demonize anyone? Can you begin to understand that the people who created this situation are also human beings doing the best they can, while at the same time acknowledging the harm done and the need to make a change?

- Is there any *action* you would like to take to change the situation, from the perspective of fierce compassion?

- Now think of a situation in your *personal life* that you strongly disagree with—a situation that was largely created by someone you know, such as a partner, child, friend, or coworker. Again, instead of just being angry about it, imagine how you would think and feel about it with a mindset of fierce compassion. Can you describe the situation in a way that does not demonize anyone? Can you begin to understand that the people who created this situation are also human beings doing the best they can, while at the same time acknowledging the harm done and the need to make a change?

- Is there any *action* you can take to try to change the situation, from a place of fierce compassion?

REFLECTION

Many people find the idea of fierce compassion liberating. It offers a way to take action and motivate change without falling into the pitfalls of anger or blame. While this is a useful ideal to pursue, it is also true that anger is a natural reaction and we will often find ourselves falling into our old reactive patterns. When this occurs, we don't need to get angry at ourselves for getting angry at others! Instead, we can have compassion for our own humanity, find our center of loving, connected presence, and try again.

21

Self-Compassion and Forgiveness

When someone has harmed us and we still feel anger and bitterness, sometimes the most compassionate thing to do is to forgive. Forgiveness involves letting go of anger at someone who has caused us harm. But forgiveness must involve grieving before letting go. The central point of forgiveness practice is that we cannot forgive others without first opening to the hurt that we have experienced. Similarly, to forgive *ourselves*, we must first open to the pain, remorse, and guilt of hurting others.

> *Forgiveness depends on being able to open to the hurt caused, whether to us or by us.*

Forgiveness doesn't mean condoning bad behavior or resuming a relationship that causes harm. If we are being harmed in a relationship, we need to protect ourselves before we can forgive. If we are harming another in a relationship, we cannot forgive ourselves if we are using this as an excuse for acting badly. We must first stop the behavior, then acknowledge and take responsibility for the harm we have caused.

At the same time, it's helpful to remember that the harm done is usually the product of a universe of interacting causes and conditions stretching back through time. We have partly inherited our temperament from our parents and grandparents, and our actions are shaped by our early childhood history, culture, health status, current events, and so forth. Therefore, we don't have complete control over precisely what we say and do from one moment to the next.

Sometimes we cause pain in life without intending it, and we may still feel sorry about causing such pain. An example is when we move across the country to start a new life, leaving friends and family behind, or when we can't give our elderly parents the attention they need because of our work situation. This kind of pain is not the fault of anyone, but it can still be acknowledged and healed with self-compassion.

The capacity to forgive requires keen awareness of our common humanity. We are all imperfect human beings whose actions stem from a web of interdependent conditions that are much larger than ourselves. In other words, we don't have to take our mistakes so personally. Paradoxically, this understanding helps us take *more* responsibility for our actions because we feel more emotionally secure. One research study asked participants to recall a recent action they felt guilty about—such as cheating on an exam, lying to a romantic partner, saying something harmful—that *still* made them feel bad about themselves when they thought about it. The researchers found that participants who were helped to be self-compassionate about their transgression reported being more motivated to apologize for the harm done, and more committed to not repeating the behavior, than those who were not helped to be self-compassionate.

> *We're imperfect human beings by nature, so there's no reason to be so unforgiving toward ourselves.*

Anneka really struggled to forgive herself after getting super angry at her friend and coworker Hilde, whom she told to f—— off. Anneka had been under a tremendous amount of pressure at work to secure a contract with new clients and was all set to close the deal at a dinner that they were hosting. The clients were pretty conservative, and Anneka knew she had to be on time and look appropriate for them to trust her. Hilde was supposed to pick her up for the dinner, but she wasn't there at the appointed time. Frantic, Anneka called her. "Where are you?" Hilde had completely forgotten about the event. "Oh, I'm so sorry," she offered lamely. Anneka dropped the f-bomb, said a few more unpleasant things, then hung up and called a taxi. Immediately afterward, Anneka felt terrible. This was her friend! Hilde hadn't done anything purposefully harmful—she simply forgot, and Anneka has been too busy to remind her. The truth was that Anneka was so anxious about closing the deal that she lost perspective and overreacted.

There are five steps to forgiveness:

1. *Opening to pain*—being present with the distress of what happened.

2. *Self-compassion*—allowing our hearts to melt with sympathy for the pain, no matter what caused it.

3. *Wisdom*—beginning to recognize that the situation wasn't entirely personal, but was the consequence of many interdependent causes and conditions.

4. *Intention to forgive*—"May I begin to forgive myself [another] for what I [he/she] did, wittingly or unwittingly, to have caused them [me] pain."

5. *Responsibility to protect*—committing ourselves to not repeat the same mistake; to stay out of harm's way, to the best of our ability.

At first Anneka harshly berated herself for her behavior, but she knew that beating up on herself wouldn't help anyone. Instead, Anneka needed to forgive herself for having made a mistake, just as everyone makes mistakes.

Anneka had learned the five steps to forgiveness from her MSC course, so she knew what to do. First, she had to accept the pain she had caused Hilde. This was really tough for Anneka, especially since she didn't get the contract she was hoping for. Her mind wanted to pin all the blame on Hilde. It was Hilde's fault! But Anneka knew the truth. There was no excuse for talking to Hilde that way. It was wrong.

Anneka allowed herself to feel in her bones what it must have been like for Hilde to hear those words—from someone she considered a friend. That took some courage because Anneka felt so bad about it. Then Anneka gave herself compassion for the pain of hurting someone she loved. "Everyone makes mistakes. I'm so sorry you wounded your friend in this manner. I know you deeply regret it." Giving herself compassion provided a bit of perspective, and Anneka was able to acknowledge the incredible stress she was under. The circumstances brought out the worst in her. Then Anneka tried to forgive herself, at least in a preliminary way, for her behavior. "May I begin to forgive myself for the pain I unwittingly inflicted on my dear friend Hilde." Anneka also made a commitment to take at least one deep breath before speaking when she felt angry. Anneka knew this might take some time because she didn't always know *when she felt angry, but she was determined to try to be less reactive when under stress.*

The next two practices will take you through the five steps to forgiveness—*forgiving others* and *forgiving ourselves.* Again, the central point of forgiveness is first opening to the hurt that we experienced or caused to others. Timing is very important because we are naturally ambivalent about feeling the guilt of hurting others or making ourselves vulnerable to being hurt again. As the saying goes, first we need to "give up all hope of a better past."

 INFORMAL PRACTICE
Forgiving Others

- Take two or three deep breaths and close your eyes for a few moments to settle and center yourself. Put your hands on your heart or use some other soothing touch as a gesture of support and self-kindness.

  Now think of a *person* who has caused you pain whom you might be ready to forgive. Then think of a *specific event* in that relationship that was mildly disturbing, perhaps a 3 on a scale of 1–10. It's important for this exercise that you choose a person and an action that you are truly ready to forgive because you realize that hanging on to anger and blame is hurting you unnecessarily. Take your time and describe the event you would like to address.

- As you do this exercise, try to make a lot of room for whatever you experience, approaching the practice with curiosity, aware of what happened without becoming swept away by the drama. If you start to feel too uncomfortable, disengage from the exercise. You can return to it anytime you like.

Opening to Pain

- Remember the details as vividly as possible, getting in touch with the pain this person caused you, perhaps even feeling it in your body.

- You only need to touch the pain, not be overwhelmed by it.

Self-Compassion

- Validate the pain, as if you were speaking to a dear friend. "*Of course* you feel this way . . . you were hurt!" "This hurts!"

- Keep giving yourself compassion, perhaps by putting a hand over your heart or elsewhere and allowing kindness to stream through your hand into your body. Or offering yourself self-compassion phrases: "May I be safe." "May I be strong." "May I be kind to myself."

- Now ask yourself, "Am I ready to forgive this person?" If not, keep giving yourself compassion.

Wisdom

- If you are *truly* ready to forgive, see if you can understand the forces that made this person act badly. Recognizing that it's only human to make mistakes, consider if there were any environmental factors that influenced what happened—factors beyond yourself and this person that you haven't taken into account.

For example, was this person under a lot of stress at the time? Or were there any difficulties that had shaped this person's personality (e.g., difficult childhood, low self-esteem, cultural factors)? Most people are just trying to live their lives the best they can. However, no matter what factors were involved, you were still hurt.

Intention to Forgive

• Now, if it feels right to forgive—and only if it feels right—begin to offer forgiveness to the other person, perhaps saying the phrase "May I begin to forgive you for what you have done, wittingly or unwittingly, that caused me pain."

Repeat this phrase two or three times.

Responsibility to Protect

• Finally, if you are ready, make a contract with yourself—deciding not to be hurt like this again, not by this person or anyone else, at least to the best of your ability.

REFLECTION

What did it feel like to reconnect with the pain you experienced? Could you offer yourself compassion? Was there any resistance?

Were you able to identify any factors you had not previously considered that led to this person's hurtful behavior? How did it feel to use the forgiveness phrase? Were you able to get in touch with feelings of resolve to protect yourself in the future?

When some people do this exercise, they discover they're just not ready to forgive. Unwillingness to forgive is itself an important learning experience. If that happened to you, try focusing on the word *begin* in the forgiveness phrase, which honors the intention without struggling to make it happen. We know we have forgiven when the heart feels free, but if forgiveness feels like a burden we aren't yet ready.

 INFORMAL PRACTICE
Forgiving Ourselves

• Take two or three deep breaths and close your eyes for a few moments to settle and center yourself. Put your hands on your heart or use some other soothing touch as a gesture of support and self-kindness.

- Now think of a person whom *you* have caused pain. Please think of a specific event that occurred in the relationship that you regret and would like to forgive yourself for. Again, choose a relatively easy situation the first time you do this exercise, perhaps a 3 on a scale of 1–10. Take your time to find the right situation to work with.

Opening to Pain

- Take a few moments to consider how your actions impacted the other person and allow yourself to feel the guilt and remorse that naturally arise when we cause someone pain. This may take some courage.

  It can help to let yourself feel the body sensations associated with guilt, making space for the physical sensations in your body.

  (If you realize that what you are feeling is shame rather than guilt, you may want to revisit the Working with Shame exercise in Chapter 17.)

Self-Compassion

- If you feel you acted wrongly, recognize that it is part of being human to make mistakes; guilt is part of the human experience.

- Offer yourself compassion for how you've suffered, perhaps by saying, "May I be kind to myself. May I accept myself as I am." If you like, put a hand on your heart or elsewhere and allow kindness to flow through your fingers into your body.

- If it feels like you need to stay here for a while, please do so. There is no need to go further.

Wisdom

- When you are ready, try to understand what led to your mistake. Take a moment to consider if any environmental factors were impacting you at the time. For instance, were you under a lot of stress? Or were certain aspects of your personality triggered in an irrational way—old buttons pushed? Take a moment to look beyond yourself and your personal interpretation of this situation.

- Or maybe you didn't actually make a mistake and were just trying to live your life in the best way you knew how?

Intention to Forgive

- Now see if you can offer forgiveness to yourself, saying the phrase "May I begin to forgive myself for what I have done, wittingly or unwittingly, that caused this person pain."

Responsibility to Protect

- And if it feels right, resolve not to hurt anyone in this manner again, at least to the best of your ability.

REFLECTION

Which was easier, forgiving *yourself* or *others*? Were you able to open to the pain of hurting another person?

Could you offer yourself compassion even though you may have felt undeserving? Did it help to identify factors that led to your behavior? How did it feel to say the forgiveness phrases? Were you able to get in touch with feelings of resolve not to hurt another in the same way again?

It takes special courage to open to the feelings of guilt and remorse that arise when we realize we have hurt someone. The more we can hold these uncomfortable feelings with compassion, the stronger will be our resolve to avoid repeating our mistake. Some people worry that forgiving ourselves will lead to abdicating responsibility for our actions. However, genuine self-forgiveness is actually a precursor to effective change.

Embracing the Good

One of the biggest benefits of self-compassion is that it doesn't just help you cope with negative emotions—it actively *generates positive emotions*. When we embrace ourselves and our experience with loving, connected presence, it feels good. It doesn't feel good in a saccharine way, nor does it resist or avoid what feels bad. Rather, self-compassion allows us to have the full range of experience, the bitter and the sweet.

Typically, however, we tend to focus much more on what's wrong than on what's right in our lives. For example, when you get an annual review at work, what do you remember the most—the points of praise or criticism? Or if you go shopping at the mall and interact with five polite salespeople and one rude one, which is most likely to stick in your mind?

The psychological term for this is *negativity bias*. Rick Hanson says the brain is like "Velcro for bad experiences and Teflon for good ones." Evolutionarily speaking, the reason we have a negativity bias is that our ancestors who fretted and worried at the end of the day—wondering where that pack of hyenas was yesterday and where

> *Focusing on the negative protected our ancestors from danger; today it leaves us with an unbalanced, unrealistic awareness.*

it might be hanging out tomorrow—were more likely to survive than our ancestors who kicked back and relaxed. This is evolutionarily adaptive when we face physical danger. However, since most of the dangers we face nowadays are threats to our sense of self, it is self-compassionate to correct the negativity bias because it distorts reality.

We need to *intentionally* recognize and absorb positive experiences to develop more realistic, balanced awareness that is not skewed toward the negative. This requires some training, just like mindfulness and self-compassion require training. Furthermore, since compassion training includes opening to pain, we may need the energy boost of focusing on positive experience to support our compassion practice.

Focusing on the positive also has important benefits. Barbara Fredrickson, who developed the "broaden-and-build" theory, posits that the evolutionary purpose of positive emotions is to broaden attention. In other words, when people feel safe and content, they become curious and start exploring their environment, noticing opportunities for food, shelter, or rest. This allows us to take advantage of opportunities that would otherwise go unnoticed.

> **When one door of happiness closes, another opens,**
> **but often we look so long at the closed door that we**
> **do not see the one that has been opened for us.**
> **—Helen Keller**

Recently there has been a movement in psychology that focuses on finding the most effective ways to help people cultivate positive emotions, and two powerful practices that have been identified are *savoring* and *gratitude*.

Savoring

Savoring involves noticing and appreciating the positive aspects of life—taking them in, letting them linger, and then letting them go. It is more than pleasure—savoring involves mindful awareness of the *experience* of pleasure. In other words, being aware that something good is happening while it's happening.

> *Savoring is mindfulness of positive experience.*

Given our natural tendency to skip over what's right and focus on what's wrong, we need to put a little extra effort into paying attention to what gives us pleasure. Luckily, savoring is simple practice—noticing the tart and juicy taste of a fresh apple, a gentle cool breeze on your cheek, the warm smile of your coworker, the hand of your partner gently holding your own. Research suggests that simply taking the time to notice and linger with these sorts of positive experiences can greatly increase our happiness.

Gratitude

Gratitude involves recognizing, acknowledging, and being grateful for the good things in our lives. If we just focus on what we want but *don't* have, we'll remain in a negative state of mind. But when we focus on what we *do* have, and give thanks for it, we radically reframe our experience.

Whereas savoring is primarily an experiential practice, gratitude is a wisdom practice. Wisdom refers to understanding how everything arises interdependently. The confluence of factors required for even a simple event to occur is mind-boggling and can inspire an attitude of awe and reverence. Gratitude involves recognizing the myriad people and events that contribute to the good in our lives. As an MSC participant once remarked, "The texture of wisdom is gratitude."

Gratitude can be aimed at the big things in life, like our health and family, but the effect of gratitude may be even more powerful when it is aimed at small things, such as when the bus arrives on time or the air conditioning is working on a hot summer day. Research shows that gratitude is also strongly linked to happiness. As the philosopher Mark Nepo wrote: "One key to knowing joy is to be easily pleased." The meditation teacher James Baraz tells this wonderful story about the power of gratitude in his book *Awakening Joy,* which we've adapted here by permission.

> *The wisdom practice called gratitude means knowing that the good in our lives arises from a multiplicity of people and events around us.*

One year I was visiting my then eighty-nine-year-old mother and brought along a magazine with an article on the beneficial effects of gratitude. As we ate dinner I told her about some of the findings. She said she was impressed by the reports but admitted she had a lifetime habit of looking at the glass half empty. "I know I'm very fortunate and have so many things to be thankful for, but little things just set me off." She said she wished she could change the habit but had doubts whether that was possible. "I'm just more used to seeing what's going wrong," she concluded.

"You know, Mom, the key to gratitude is really in the way we frame a situation," I began. "For instance, suppose all of a sudden your television isn't getting good reception."

"That's a scenario I can relate to," she agreed with a knowing smile.

"One way to describe your experience would be to say, 'This is so annoying I could scream!' Or you could say, 'This is so annoying . . . and my life is really very blessed.'" She agreed that could make a big difference.

"But I don't think I can remember to do that," she sighed.

So together we made up a gratitude game to remind her. Each time she complained about something, I would simply say "and . . . ," to which she would respond "and my life is very blessed." I was elated to see that she was willing to try it out. Although it had started as just a fun game, after a while it began to have some real impact. Her mood grew brighter as our weeks became filled with gratitude. To my delight and amazement, my mother has continued doing the practice, and the change has been revolutionary.

 INFORMAL PRACTICE
Sense and Savor Walk

This savoring practice is particularly uplifting when it takes place in a beautiful natural setting, such as a garden or in the woods, but it can be practiced most anywhere that you do not feel self-conscious.

- Set aside 15 minutes to amble about outdoors. The purpose of the walk is to notice and savor any attractive objects or positive internal experiences, slowly, one after another, using all your senses—sight, smell, sound, touch . . . maybe even taste.

- The goal is not to "try" to enjoy yourself or to make anything happen. Just *allow* yourself to notice, be drawn into, linger with, and then let go of whatever gives you pleasure—whatever calls to you.

- How many beautiful, attractive, or inspiring things do you notice while you're walking? Do you enjoy the scent of pine, the warm sun, a beautiful leaf, the shape of a stone, a smiling face, the song of a bird, the feeling of the earth under your feet?

- When you find something delightful or pleasant, let yourself be drawn into it. Really savor it. Smell the freshly cut grass or feel the texture of a stick, if you like. *Give yourself over* to the experience as if it were the only thing that existed in the world.

- When you lose interest and would like to discover something new, let it go and wait until you discover something else that is attractive and delightful to you. Be like a bumblebee going from flower to flower. When you are full with one, go to another.

- Take your time, move slowly, and see what comes.

REFLECTION

How did it feel to selectively attend to positive experiences? Did you notice anything that you might have ordinarily overlooked? Were you able to linger with and absorb pleasure and beauty?

How are you feeling now compared to before you did this practice?

Most people find that letting themselves soak in positive experience also makes them happier. This exercise can also reveal how our mental chatter *about* our experience interferes with enjoying it. When we refocus on our direct experience of beauty, however, our senses are enhanced such that colors become brighter, sounds become clearer, smells more aromatic, and so on. As Emily Dickinson wrote, "To live is so startling, it leaves little room for other occupations."

INFORMAL PRACTICE
Savoring Food

Savoring food is mindful eating with the added invitation to *enjoy* the experience of eating.

- Select a snack or a meal that you would like to eat.

- Take a moment and enjoy how good the food looks to you. Then savor the smell and how the food feels to the touch.

- Begin to reflect on the many hands that were involved in bringing this food to your mouth—the farmer, the trucker, the grocer . . .

- Now eat *very slowly*, noticing first how you may be salivating before reaching for the food, bringing it to your mouth, noticing when it crosses your lips, when you bite down, whether there is a splash of flavor, when you begin to swallow . . .

- Continue eating in this way, giving yourself full permission to enjoy every moment of the experience of eating, as if it were the first and last meal of your life.

- When you are done, notice the "finish"—how the flavors linger in your mouth.

REFLECTION

Did the food taste different when you gave yourself permission to take your time and enjoy it? What was it like to eat in this manner?

Savoring food usually brings immediate satisfaction and well-being. Ironically, when we eat mindlessly, we usually don't enjoy our food at all, and often overeat. Research shows that an additional benefit of mindful eating is that it helps us to maintain our weight and stop eating when we're full.

EXERCISE

Gratitude for the Big and Small Things

Write down five *big things* in your life that are very important to you and that you are grateful for. Examples are your health, your children, your career, your friends.

1. _____

2. _____

3. _____

4. _____

5. _____

Now write down five *small and insignificant things* in your life—things you usually overlook—that you are grateful for. Examples are buttons, a bicycle tire pump, warm water, a genuine smile, reading glasses.

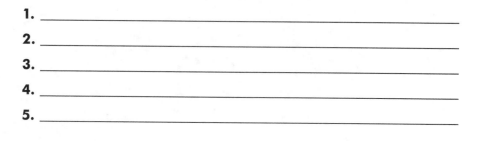

1. _____

2. _____

3. _____

4. _____

5. _____

REFLECTION

Did anything show up on your list that surprised you? Was it easier to feel grati-tude for the big things or the small things? How do you feel after this exercise, compared to before?

You can do this practice when you wake up in the morning and before you get out of bed, or in the evening after you turn out the lights and before you fall asleep. Try using the five fingers on each hand—five for the big things and five for the small things that you are grateful for. It takes only a few minutes, but research shows that "counting your blessings" can have a big impact on your mental health.

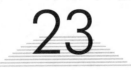

23

Self-Appreciation

Most people recognize the importance of expressing gratitude and appreciation toward others. But what about ourselves? That one doesn't come so easily.

The negativity bias is especially strong toward ourselves. Self-appreciation not only feels unnatural—it can feel downright wrong. Because our tendency is to focus on our inadequacies rather than appreciate our strengths, we often have a skewed perspective of who we are. Think about it. When you receive a compliment, do you take it in, or does it bounce off you almost immediately? We usually feel uncomfortable just *thinking* about our good qualities. The counterargument immediately arises: "I'm not always that way" or "I have a lot of bad qualities too." Again, this reaction demonstrates the negativity bias because when we receive unpleasant feedback, our first thoughts are not typically "Yes, but I'm not *always* that way" or "Are you aware of all my *good* qualities?"

> *Most of us feel it's simply wrong to appreciate ourselves.*

Many of us are actually afraid to acknowledge our own goodness. Some common reasons given for this are:

- I don't want to alienate my friends by being arrogant.

- My good qualities are not a problem that needs to be fixed, so I don't need to focus on them.

- I'm afraid I would be putting myself on a pedestal, only to fall off.

- It will make me feel superior and separate from others.

Of course, there is a big difference between simply acknowledging what's true—that we have good as well as not-so-good qualities—and saying that we're perfect or better than others. It's important to appreciate our strengths as well as have compassion for our weaknesses so that we embrace the whole of ourselves, exactly as we are.

We can apply the three components of self-compassion—self-kindness, common humanity, and mindfulness—to our positive qualities as well as our negative ones. These three factors together allow us to appreciate ourselves in a healthy and balanced way.

Self-Appreciation

Self-Kindness: Part of being kind to ourselves involves expressing appreciation for our good qualities, just as we would do with a good friend.

Common Humanity: When we remember that having good qualities is part of being human, we can acknowledge our strengths without feeling isolated or better than others.

Mindfulness: To appreciate ourselves, we need to pay attention to our good qualities rather than taking them for granted.

It's important to recognize that the practice of self-appreciation is not selfish or self-centered. Rather, it simply recognizes that good qualities are part of being human. Although some children may have been raised with the belief that humility means *not* recognizing their accomplishments, that approach can harm children's self-concept and get in the way of knowing themselves properly. Self-appreciation is a way to correct our negativity bias toward ourselves and see ourselves more clearly as a whole person. Self-appreciation also provides the emotional resilience and self-confidence needed to give to others.

Being human includes good as well as bad qualities, so self-appreciation is realistic, not selfish.

The best-selling author and spiritual teacher Marianne Williamson writes, "We are all meant to shine, as children do. . . . And as we let our own light shine, we unconsciously give other people permission to do the same. As we are liberated from our own fear, our presence automatically liberates others."

When we honor ourselves, we also honor all those who have helped nurture and support us along the way.

Wisdom and gratitude are central to self-appreciation as well. These qualities, discussed in the previous chapter, help us to see our good qualities in a broader context. When we appreciate ourselves, we're also appreciating all the causes, conditions, and people—including friends, parents, and teachers—who helped us develop those good qualities in the first place. This means we don't need to take our own good qualities so personally!

Alice grew up in a stern Protestant family where humility and self-effacement were the expected norm. When she was eight years old and came home with a trophy for winning her third-grade spelling bee, she remembers, her mother just raised her eyebrows and said, "Now don't you be getting too big for your britches." Every time Alice accomplished anything she felt she had to downplay it or else receive the disapproval of her family.

Later on in life, Alice started dating a man named Theo who thought she was beautiful and kind and smart and wonderful and liked to tell her so. Alice would not only cringe with embarrassment; Theo's comments made her anxious. What if Theo finds out I'm not perfect? What happens if I let him down? She would continually brush aside his comments when he said something nice, leaving Theo feeling perplexed and on the other side of an invisible wall.

Alice was becoming adept at self-compassion, especially the capacity to see her personal inadequacies as part of common humanity. Self-appreciation made sense to Alice, primarily conceptually, but she knew she had a way to go. First Alice made a mental note of everything good that she did during the day—a moment of kindness, a success, a small accomplishment. Then she tried to say something appreciative about it, such as "That was well done, Alice." When Alice spoke to herself like this, she felt like she was violating an invisible contract from childhood and it made her uneasy, but she persisted. "I'm not saying I'm better than anyone else or that I'm perfect. I'm simply acknowledging that this too is true." Eventually Alice made a commitment to take in and savor the heartfelt compliments Theo gave her. Theo was so delighted by this turn of events that he bought her a bracelet that said on the inside, I may not be perfect, but parts of me are excellent!

EXERCISE

How Do I Relate to My Good Qualities?

Consider the following questions, being as candid and honest as possible.

- How do you react to compliments? Do you receive them happily or graciously, or do you tense up, avoid, or dismiss them?

- In your private moments, do you find it comfortable or uncomfortable to appreciate your good qualities?

- If you find that it's uncomfortable to appreciate your good qualities, consider why that might be so. Are you afraid of becoming arrogant, falling off the pedestal, becoming complacent, or feeling separate from others, or is there some other reason? How is it for you?

REFLECTION

Many people find that the edge of their practice is self-appreciation rather than self-compassion. Somehow it's okay to accept one's flaws and inadequacies, but to acknowledge one's strengths and accomplishments? Yuck! If this is you, it means that you may really benefit from making self-appreciation a conscious practice in your daily life.

 EXERCISE
Self-Appreciation

This exercise will help you discover qualities that you appreciate about yourself, especially by acknowledging influences in your life that helped you develop these good qualities.

If you experience any uneasiness during this exercise, make some space for whatever you're feeling and let yourself be just as you are.

- Take two or three deep breaths and close your eyes for a few moments to settle and center yourself. Put your hands on your heart or use some other soothing touch as a gesture of support and self-kindness.

- Now think of three to five things you appreciate about yourself. The first few things that come to mind may be somewhat superficial. See if you can open to what you *really*, deep down, like and appreciate about yourself. Please take your time and be honest.

- Now consider each of these positive qualities, one by one, and offer yourself an inner nod of appreciation for having these gifts.

- Notice if you feel any discomfort as you think about your good qualities and make space for that, allowing your experience to be just as it is. Remember that you aren't saying you *always* show these good qualities or that you're better than others. You're simply acknowledging that this, too, is true.

- Now consider, are there any people who helped you develop your good qualities? Maybe friends, parents, teachers, even authors of books who had a positive impact on you?

- Think about each one of these positive influences and send each one some gratitude and appreciation as well.

- Let yourself savor, just for this moment, feeling good about yourself—let it really soak in.

REFLECTION

Were you able to think of some good qualities? How did it feel when you gave yourself appreciation? Did self-appreciation become easier when you brought in gratitude and appreciation for others?

The interesting part of this exercise for most people is how much easier it is to accept our good qualities when we realize how intertwined they are with the lives and contributions of others. Shining the light of appreciation on ourselves seems less self-focused, and we feel less alone, when we include others in the circle of appreciation.

Quite a lot of people find this practice difficult, especially those who suffered from childhood trauma or were raised in an environment where it was

"bad" to feel proud of their achievements. Sometimes when we try to appreciate our good qualities, we recall how our good qualities were *not* appreciated,
or our not-so-good qualities become more apparent to us. That's backdraft
(see Chapter 8). If this happened to you, remember that backdraft is part of
the transformation process, and be tender and compassionate with yourself.
Backdraft may also be a signal that this is a fruitful practice for you, to be done
slowly, with patience. When you give yourself permission to acknowledge your
whole self—the good as well as the bad—you open the door to living a fuller,
more authentic life.

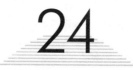

24

Taking It Forward

This workbook is coming to an end, and you have learned a wide array of principles and practices for cultivating self-compassion. You might be wondering how to integrate what you have learned into your daily life and how to continue practicing for the coming months, even years.

The question is sometimes raised, "What is the right practice for me?" The best answer comes from meditation teacher Sharon Salzberg: "The one you are most committed to!" We only discover in hindsight which practices we are most committed to, but a good start is probably the practices that were easiest and *most enjoyable*. What are they? You will have a chance to reflect on that below.

> *The best practice for you is the one you're most committed to.*

It is also good to know which practices were especially *meaningful* or *helpful* to you. Perhaps you bumped up against a growth edge and had some backdraft, but you sense that there is freedom just around the corner. If so, you can make a note of that and return to the practice when you feel ready to do so, all the while being self-compassionate about *how* you practice.

Here are some tips for maintaining a practice:

◇ Make your practice as pleasant as possible so it is self-reinforcing.

◇ Start small—short practices can make a big difference.

◇ Practice during daily life, when you need it the most.

◇ Be compassionate when your practice lapses, and just start again.

◇ Let go of unnecessary effort to practice in the right way—just be warm and friendly with yourself.

✧ Pick a consistent time to practice each day

✧ Identify obstacles to practice

✧ Read books on mindfulness and self-compassion

✧ Journal about your practice experiences

✧ Stay connected—practice in community

✧ Listen to guided meditations, available using the links in this workbook

✧ Take the MSC program. The Center for Mindful Self-Compassion (*www.centerformsc.org*) has a directory of MSC courses offered worldwide, as well as online MSC training.

EXERCISE

What Would I Like to Remember?

Before you finish this book, you might want to reflect on all you learned. You might also feel overwhelmed by the sheer volume of new learning. Therefore, the question arises, "What would I like to remember?" Please answer the following two questions—one of which is a heart question and the other a practical question.

Heart Question

- Close your eyes for a moment and allow yourself to reflect on your experience while going through this workbook. Scanning the terrain of your heart, *feeling* your heart, ask yourself, "What touched me, moved me, or shifted inside of me?" To support your memory, you can also review any notes you may have made in this book or in a separate notebook.

  It could be anything, really—perhaps a surprise, a realization, or an insight? Or maybe something that comforted you, challenged you, uplifted you, or transformed you along the way?

  Take your time and write down what arises in your mind—what you would like to remember.

Practical Question

- Next, write down any *practices* that you might like to remember and repeat, going forward. See if there are some formal meditations that you found helpful and also some informal practices for daily life. To help you recall the practices, flip through this workbook, particularly noting the practices that you resonated with most easily or that had the most powerful impact on you.

A FINAL WORD

We are sincerely grateful to you, our readers, for joining us on this path of mindfulness and self-compassion. We know that it requires courage and commitment to open to the fullness of our human experience. Hopefully your efforts have already borne fruit, perhaps in the form of a lighter, happier heart. The practice is paradoxical that way—the more we dip into suffering with mindfulness and compassion, the more it frees the heart. We must be patient, though.

The practice of mindfulness and self-compassion is a lifelong journey—we never arrive. This is a good thing because it renders each moment of our lives more precious, realizing each moment is an opportunity to practice. We especially appreciate the opportunity to practice together, in community. We hope that you consider yourself part of this growing community in a way that nourishes you.

In closing, may the fruits of our common efforts be dedicated to *all* beings, and may we never forget to include ourselves in the great circle of compassion.

Resources

BOOKS

Baraz, J., & Alexander, S. (2012). *Awakening joy.* Berkeley, CA: Parallax Press.

Bluth, K. (2017). *The self-compassion workbook for teens.* Oakland, CA: New Harbinger Press.

Brach, T. (2003). *Radical acceptance: Embracing your life with the heart of a Buddha.* New York: Bantam.

Brach, T. (2013). *True refuge.* New York: Bantam Books.

Brown, B. (2010). *The gifts of imperfection.* Center City, MN: Hazelden.

Brown, B. (2012). *Daring greatly.* New York: Penguin.

Chödrön, P. (1997). *When things fall apart: Heart advice for difficult times.* Boston: Shambhala.

Chödrön, P. (2005). *Start where you are: How to accept yourself and others.* London: Element/HarperCollins.

Dalai Lama. (1995). *The power of compassion.* New York: HarperCollins.

Fredrickson, B. (2013). *Love 2.0.* New York: Hudson Street Press.

Germer, C. K. (2009). *The mindful path to self-compassion.* New York: Guilford Press.

Germer, C., & Neff, K. (in press). *Teaching the Mindful Self-Compassion program: A guide for professionals.* New York: Guilford Press.

Gilbert, P. (2009). *The compassionate mind.* Oakland, CA: New Harbinger Press.

Hanh, T. N. (1998). *Teaching on love.* Berkeley, CA: Parallax Press.

Hanson, R. (2009). *The Buddha's brain.* Oakland, CA: New Harbinger Press.

Hanson, R. (2014). *Hardwiring happiness.* New York: Harmony/Crown.

Jinpa, T. (2015). *A fearless heart.* New York: Avery/Penguin.

Kabat-Zinn, J. (1990). *Full catastrophe living.* New York: Dell.

Keltner, D. (2009). *Born to be good.* New York: Norton.

Kornfield, J. (1993). *A path with heart.* New York: Bantam Books.

Neff, K. (2011). *Self-compassion: The proven power of being kind to yourself.* New York: William Morrow.

Rosenberg, M. (2003). *Nonviolent communication: A language of life.* Encinitas, CA: PuddleDancer Press.

Salzberg, S. (1997). *Lovingkindness: The revolutionary art of happiness.* Boston: Shambhala.

Salzberg, S. (2008). *The kindness handbook.* Boulder, CO: Sounds True.

Siegel, D. J. (2010). *Mindsight.* New York: Bantam.

ONLINE AND AUDIO COURSES BY KRISTIN NEFF AND CHRISTOPHER GERMER

The power of self compassion: A step-by-step training to bring kindness and inner strength to any moment of your life. Sounds True, *www.soundstrue.com.* Eight-week online training course by Kristin Neff and Christopher Germer.

Self-compassion: Step by step: The proven power of being kind to yourself. Sounds True. *www.soundstrue.com.* Six-session audio training course by Kristin Neff.

WEBSITES BY KRISTIN NEFF AND CHRISTOPHER GERMER

Center for Mindful Self-Compassion
www.centerformsc.org
- Audio and video recordings by Christopher Germer and Kristin Neff
- Resources for supporting continuing practice
- Online offerings for continuing study
- Information about upcoming retreats, workshops, and other activities related to self-compassion
- A searchable database of MSC teachers and programs worldwide

Social Media
- Facebook page at *www.facebook.com/centerformsc*
- Twitter at *@centerformsc*

Kristin Neff
www.self-compassion.org
- Video presentations
- Guided meditations
- Self-compassion exercises
- Testing your own self-compassion level
- Huge library of self-compassion research
- Information about upcoming talks and workshops

Social Media
- Facebook page at *www.facebook.com/selfcompassion*
- Twitter at *@self_compassion*

Christopher Germer
www.chrisgermer.com
- Guided meditations
- Information about upcoming talks and workshops

Social Media
- Facebook page at *www.facebook.com/Christopher-K-Germer-PhD-The-Mindful-Path-to-Self-Compassion-141943624277*

OTHER HELPFUL WEBSITES

Acceptance and Commitment Therapy
www.contextualscience.org/act

Center for Compassion and Altruism Research and Education, Stanford Medicine
www.ccare.stanford.edu

Center for Healthy Minds, University of Wisconsin–Madison
www.centerhealthyminds.org

Center for Mindfulness and Compassion, Cambridge Health Alliance, Harvard Medical School Teaching Hospital
www.chacmc.org

Center for Mindfulness in Medicine, Health Care, and Society, University of Massachusetts Medical School
www.umassmed.edu/cfm

Cognitively-Based Compassion Training, Emory University
www.tibet.emory.edu/cognitively-based-compassion-training

Compassion Cultivation Training and Contemplative Education, Compassion Institute
www.compassioninstitute.com

Compassion Focused Therapy, Compassionate Mind Foundation
www.compassionatemind.co.uk

Greater Good Magazine, Greater Good Science Center at UC Berkeley
www.greatergood.berkeley.edu

Institute for Meditation and Psychotherapy
www.meditationandpsychotherapy.org

Internal Family Systems, Center for Self Leadership
www.selfleadership.org

Mindfulness-Based Cognitive Therapy
www.mbct.com

Notes

INTRODUCTION

PAGE 1: **Our task is not to seek for love:** Quote retrieved from *www.bbc.co.uk/worldservice/learningenglish/movingwords/quotefeature/rumi.shtml*.

... **self-compassionate tend to have greater happiness, life satisfaction:** Zessin, U., Dickhauser, O., & Garbade, S. (2015). The relationship between self-compassion and well-being: A meta-analysis. *Applied Psychology: Health and Well-Being, 7*(3), 340–364.

... **and motivation:** Breines, J. G., & Chen, S. (2012). Self-compassion increases self-improvement motivation. *Personality and Social Psychology Bulletin, 38*(9), 1133–1143.

... **better relationships:** Neff, K. D., & Beretvas, S. N. (2013). The role of self-compassion in romantic relationships. *Self and Identity, 12*(1), 78–98.

... **and physical health:** Dunne, S., Sheffield, D., & Chilcot, J. (2016). Brief report: Self-compassion, physical health and the mediating role of health-promoting behaviours. *Journal of Health Psychology*.

... **and less anxiety and depression:** MacBeth, A., & Gumley, A. (2012). Exploring compassion: A meta-analysis of the association between self-compassion and psychopathology. *Clinical Psychology Review, 32*, 545–552.

... **stressful life events such as divorce:** Sbarra, D. A., Smith, H. L., & Mehl, M. R. (2012). When leaving your ex, love yourself: Observational ratings of self-compassion predict the course of emotional recovery following marital separation. *Psychological Science, 23*, 261–269.

... **health crises:** Brion, J. M., Leary, M. R., & Drabkin, A. S. (2014). Self-compassion and reactions to serious illness: The case of HIV. *Journal of Health Psychology, 19*(2), 218–229.

PAGE 1:   . . . **academic failure:** Neff, K. D., Hseih, Y., & Dejitthirat, K. (2005). Self-compassion, achievement goals, and coping with academic failure. *Self and Identity, 4,* 263–287.

. . . **even combat trauma:** Hiraoka, R., Meyer, E. C., Kimbrel, N. A., DeBeer, B. B., Gulliver, S. B., & Morissette, S. B. (2015). Self-compassion as a prospective predictor of PTSD symptom severity among trauma-exposed U.S. Iraq and Afghanistan war veterans. *Journal of Traumatic Stress, 28,* 1–7.

PAGE 2:   . . . **training programs such as mindfulness-based stress reduction:** Birnie, K., Speca, M., & Carlson, L. E. (2010). Exploring self-compassion and empathy in the context of mindfulness-based stress reduction (MBSR). *Stress and Health, 26,* 359–371.

. . . **and mindfulness-based cognitive therapy:** Kuyken, W., Watkins, E., Holden, E., White, K., Taylor, R. S., Byford, S., et al. (2010). How does mindfulness-based cognitive therapy work? *Behavior Research and Therapy, 48,* 1105–1112.

. . . **also increase self-compassion:** Keng, S., Smoski, M. J., Robins, C. J., Ekblad, A. G., & Brantley, J. G. (2012). Mechanisms of change in mindfulness-based stress reduction: Self-compassion and mindfulness as mediators of intervention outcomes. *Journal of Cognitive Psychotherapy, 26*(3), 270–280.

. . . **increases in self-compassion and mindfulness, reduces anxiety and depression:** Neff, K. D., & Germer, C. K. (2013). A pilot study and randomized controlled trial of the Mindful Self-Compassion program. *Journal of Clinical Psychology, 69*(1), 28–44.

. . . **enhances overall well-being:** Bluth, K., Gaylord, S. A., Campo, R. A., Mullarkey, M. C., & Hobbs, L. (2016). Making friends with yourself: A mixed methods pilot study of a Mindful Self-Compassion program for adolescents. *Mindfulness, 7*(2), 1–14.

. . . **and even stabilizes glucose levels among people with diabetes:** Friis, A. M., Johnson, M. H., Cutfield, R. G., & Consedine, N. S. (2016). Kindness matters: A randomized controlled trial of a mindful self-compassion intervention improves depression, distress, and HbA1c among patients with diabetes. *Diabetes Care, 39*(11), 1963–1971.

PAGE 3:   **Though it's beneficial to feel good about ourselves:** Neff, K. D., & Vonk, R. (2009). Self-compassion versus global self-esteem: Two different ways of relating to oneself. *Journal of Personality, 77,* 23–50.

. . . **publication of *Mindfulness and Psychotherapy:*** Germer, C. K., Siegel, R., & Fulton, P. (Eds.). (2013). *Mindfulness and psychotherapy* (2nd ed.). New York: Guilford Press.

PAGE 4:   **In 2009, I published *The Mindful Path to Self-Compassion:*** Germer, C. K. (2009). *The mindful path to self-compassion: Freeing yourself from destructive thoughts and emotions.* New York: Guilford Press.

The following year, Kristin published *Self-Compassion:* Neff, K. D. (2011). *Self-compassion: The proven power of being kind to yourself.* New York: William Morrow.

PAGE 5: **. . . the MSC professional training manual, to be published by The Guilford Press:** Germer, C. K., & Neff, K. D. (in press). *Teaching the Mindful Self-Compassion program: A guide for professionals.* New York: Guilford Press.

CHAPTER 1
What Is Self-Compassion?

PAGE 10: **. . . self-kindness, common humanity, and mindfulness:** Neff, K. D. (2003). Self-compassion: An alternative conceptualization of a healthy attitude toward oneself. *Self and Identity, 2,* 85–102.

PAGE 14: **. . . 16% are about equal:** Knox, M., Neff, K., & Davidson, O. (2016, June). *Comparing compassion for self and others: Impacts on personal and interpersonal well-being.* Paper presented at the 14th annual meeting of the Association for Contextual Behavioral Science World Conference, Seattle, WA.

CHAPTER 2
What Self-Compassion Is Not

PAGE 20: **. . . likely to engage in perspective taking:** Neff, K. D., & Pommier, E. (2013). The relationship between self-compassion and other-focused concern among college undergraduates, community adults, and practicing meditators. *Self and Identity, 12*(2), 160–176.

. . . ruminate on how bad things are: Raes, F. (2010). Rumination and worry as mediators of the relationship between self-compassion and depression and anxiety. *Personality and Individual Differences, 48,* 757–761.

. . . cope with tough situations like divorce: Sbarra, D. A., Smith, H. L., & Mehl, M. R. (2012). When leaving your ex, love yourself: Observational ratings of self-compassion predict the course of emotional recovery following marital separation. *Psychological Science, 23,* 261–269.

. . . trauma: Hiraoka, R., Meyer, E. C., Kimbrel, N. A., DeBeer, B. B., Gulliver, S. B., & Morissette, S. B. (2015). Self-compassion as a prospective predictor of PTSD symptom severity among trauma-exposed U.S. Iraq and Afghanistan war veterans. *Journal of Traumatic Stress, 28,* 1–7.

. . . or chronic pain: Wren, A. A., Somers, T. J., Wright, M. A., Goetz, M. C., Leary, M. R., Fras, A. M., et al. (2012). Self-compassion in patients with persistent musculoskeletal pain: Relationship of self-compassion to adjustment to persistent pain. *Journal of Pain and Symptom Management, 43*(4), 759–770.

PAGE 20: . . . **caring and supportive in romantic relationships:** Neff, K. D., & Beretvas, S. N. (2013). The role of self-compassion in romantic relationships. *Self and Identity, 12*(1), 78–98.

. . . **more likely to compromise in relationship conflicts:** Yarnell, L. M., & Neff, K. D. (2013). Self-compassion, interpersonal conflict resolutions, and well-being. *Self and Identity, 2*(2), 146–159.

. . . **more compassionate and forgiving toward others:** Neff, K. D., & Pommier, E. (2013). The relationship between self-compassion and other-focused concern among college undergraduates, community adults, and practicing meditators. *Self and Identity, 12*(2), 160–176.

PAGE 21: . . . **healthier behaviors like exercise:** Magnus, C. M. R., Kowalski, K. C., & McHugh, T. L. F. (2010). The role of self-compassion in women's self-determined motives to exercise and exercise-related outcomes. *Self and Identity, 9*, 363–382.

. . . **eating well:** Schoenefeld, S. J., & Webb, J. B. (2013). Self-compassion and intuitive eating in college women: Examining the contributions of distress tolerance and body image acceptance and action. *Eating Behaviors, 14*(4), 493–496.

. . . **drinking less:** Brooks, M., Kay-Lambkin, F., Bowman, J., & Childs, S. (2012). Self-compassion amongst clients with problematic alcohol use. *Mindfulness, 3*(4), 308–317.

. . . **going to the doctor more regularly:** Terry, M. L., Leary, M. R., Mehta, S., & Henderson, K. (2013). Self-compassionate reactions to health threats. *Personality and Social Psychology Bulletin, 39*(7), 911–926.

. . . **take greater personal responsibility for their actions:** Zhang, J. W., & Chen, S. (2016). Self-compassion promotes personal improvement from regret experiences via acceptance. *Personality and Social Psychology Bulletin, 42*(2), 244–258.

. . . **more likely to apologize if they've offended someone:** Howell, A. J., Dopko, R. L., Turowski, J. B., & Buro, K. (2011). The disposition to apologize. *Personality and Individual Differences, 51*(4), 509–514.

. . . **don't beat themselves up when they fail:** Neff, K. D. (2003). Development and validation of a scale to measure self-compassion. *Self and Identity, 2*, 223–250.

. . . **less afraid of failure:** Neff, K. D., Hseih, Y., & Dejitthirat, K. (2005). Self-compassion, achievement goals, and coping with academic failure. *Self and Identity, 4*, 263–287.

. . . **more likely to try again and to persist in their efforts after failing:** Breines, J. G., & Chen, S. (2012). Self-compassion increases self-improvement motivation. *Personality and Social Psychology Bulletin, 38*(9), 1133–1143.

PAGE 22: **Compared with self-esteem, self-compassion is less contingent:** Neff, K. D., & Vonk, R. (2009). Self-compassion versus global self-esteem: Two different ways of relating to oneself. *Journal of Personality, 77*, 23–50.

CHAPTER 3
The Benefits of Self-Compassion

PAGE 25:   **People who are more self-compassionate experience greater well-being:**

MacBeth, A., & Gumley, A. (2012). Exploring compassion: A meta-analysis of the association between self-compassion and psychopathology. *Clinical Psychology Review, 32,* 545–552.

Zessin, U., Dickhauser, O., & Garbade, S. (2015). The relationship between self-compassion and well-being: A meta-analysis. *Applied Psychology: Health and Well-Being, 7*(3), 340–364.

Neff, K. D., Long, P., Knox, M. C., Davidson, O., Kuchar, A., Costigan, A., et al. (in press). The forest and the trees: Examining the association of self-compassion and its positive and negative components with psychological functioning. *Self and Identity.*

Hall, C. W., Row, K. A., Wuensch, K. L., & Godley, K. R. (2013). The role of self-compassion in physical and psychological well-being. *Journal of Psychology, 147*(4), 311–323.

. . . **people who took the MSC course:** Neff, K. D., & Germer, C. K. (2013). A pilot study and randomized controlled trial of the Mindful Self-Compassion program. *Journal of Clinical Psychology, 69*(1), 28–44.

PAGE 27:   **The Self-Compassion Scale measures:** Neff, K. D. (2003). Development and validation of a scale to measure self-compassion. *Self and Identity, 2,* 223–250.

. . . **adapted version of the short form:** Raes, F., Pommier, E., Neff, K. D., & Van Gucht, D. (2011). Construction and factorial validation of a short form of the Self-Compassion Scale. *Clinical Psychology and Psychotherapy, 18,* 250–255.

PAGE 29:   **Journaling is an effective way to express emotions:** Ullrich, P. M., & Lutgendorf, S. K. (2002). Journaling about stressful events: Effects of cognitive processing and emotional expression. *Annals of Behavioral Medicine, 24*(3), 244–250.

CHAPTER 4
The Physiology of Self-Criticism and Self-Compassion

PAGE 31:   . . . **created compassion-focused therapy:** Gilbert, P. (2009). *The compassionate mind.* London: Constable.

The threat-defense system evolved: LeDoux, J. E. (2003). *Synaptic self: How our brains become who we are.* New York: Penguin.

. . . **the mammalian care system evolved:** Solomon, J., & George, C. (1996). Defining the caregiving system: Toward a theory of caregiving. *Infant Mental Health Journal, 17*(3), 183–197.

PAGE 31:   **Two reliable ways of activating the care system** . . . Stellar, J. E., & Keltner, D. (2014). Compassion. In M. Tugade, L. Shiota, & L. Kirby (Eds.), *Handbook of positive emotions* (pp. 329–341). New York: Guilford Press.

PAGE 32:   **. . . researchers asked participants to imagine receiving compassion:** Rockcliff, H., Gilbert, P., McEwan, K., Lightman, S., & Glover, D. (2008). A pilot exploration of heart rate variability and salivary cortisol responses to compassion-focused imagery. *Clinical Neuropsychiatry, 5,* 132–139.

CHAPTER 5
The Yin and Yang of Self-Compassion

PAGE 38:   **. . . traditional feminine gender role norms:** Eagly, A. H. (1987). *Sex differences in social behavior: A social-role interpretation.* Hillsdale, NJ: Erlbaum.

CHAPTER 6
Mindfulness

PAGE 44:   **. . . "awareness of present-moment experience with acceptance":** Bishop, S. R., Lau, M., Shapiro, S., Carlson, L., Anderson, N. D., Carmody, J., et al. (2004). Mindfulness: A proposed operational definition. *Clinical Psychology Science and Practice, 11,* 191–206.

PAGE 45:   **. . .** *the default mode network:* Raichle, M. E., MacLeod, A. M., Snyder, A. Z., Powers, W. J., Gusnard, D. A., & Shulman, G. L. (2001). A default mode of brain function. *Proceedings of the National Academy of Sciences of the USA, 98*(2), 676–682.

PAGE 46:   **. . . deactivate the default mode network:** Brewer, J. A., Worhunsky, P. D., Gray, J. R., Tang, Y. Y., Weber, J., & Kober, H. (2011). Meditation experience is associated with differences in default mode network activity and connectivity. *Proceedings of the National Academy of Sciences of the USA, 108*(50), 20254–20259.

    . . . during our normal activities: Taylor, V. A., Daneault, V., Grant, J., Scavone, G., Breton, E., Roffe-Vidal, S., et al. (2013). Impact of meditation training on the default mode network during a restful state. *Social Cognitive and Affective Neuroscience, 8*(1), 4–14.

CHAPTER 7
Letting Go of Resistance

PAGE 51:   **Suffering = Pain × Resistance:** Young, S. (2016). *A pain processing algorithm.* Retrieved February 8, 2018, from *www.shinzen.org/wp-content/uploads/2016/12/art_painprocessingalg.pdf.*

. . . just makes the pain more intense: McCracken, L. M., & Eccleston, C. (2003). Coping or acceptance: What to do about chronic pain? *Pain, 105*(1), 197–204.

. . . when we try to suppress our unwanted thoughts or feelings: Wegner, D. M., Schneider, D. J., Carter, S. R., & White, T. L. (1987). Paradoxical effects of thought suppression. *Journal of Personality and Social Psychology, 53*(1), 5–13.

CHAPTER 8
Backdraft

PAGE 57: . . . we may reexperience old pain as it starts to be released: Germer, C. K., & Neff, K. D. (2013). Self-compassion in clinical practice. *Journal of Clinical Psychology, 69*(8), 856–867.

PAGE 59: . . . this practice can help regulate strong emotions such as anger: Singh, N. N., Wahler, R. G., Adkins, A. D., Myers, R. E., & the Mindfulness Research Group. (2003). Soles of the feet: A mindfulness-based self-control intervention for aggression by an individual with mild mental retardation and mental illness. *Research in Developmental Disabilities, 24,* 158–169.

CHAPTER 9
Developing Loving-Kindness

PAGE 64: . . . the Pali term *metta:* Salzberg, S. (1997). *Lovingkindness: The revolutionary art of happiness.* Boston: Shambhala.

". . . deep desire to alleviate that suffering": Goetz, J. L., Keltner, D., & Simon-Thomas, E. (2010). Compassion: An evolutionary analysis and empirical review. *Psychological Bulletin, 136,* 351–374.

According to the Dalai Lama: Dalai Lama. (2003). *Lighting the path: The Dalai Lama teaches on wisdom and compassion.* South Melbourne, Australia: Thomas C. Lothian.

PAGE 65: . . . loving-kindness meditation is "dose dependent": Pace, T. W. W., Negi, L. T., Adame, D. D., Cole, S. P., Sivilli, T. I., Brown, T. D., et al. (2009). Effect of compassion meditation on neuroendocrine, innate immune and behavioral responses to psychosocial stress. *Psychoneuroendocrinology, 43*(1), 87–98.

. . . reduced negative emotions like anxiety and depression: Shonin, E., Van Gordon, W., Compare, A., Zangeneh, M., & Griffiths, M. D. (2014). Buddhist-derived loving-kindness and compassion meditation for the treatment of psychopathology: A systematic review. *Mindfulness, 6,* 1161–1180.

. . . increased positive emotions like happiness and joy: Fredrickson, B. L., Cohn, M. A., Coffey, K. A., Pek, J., & Finkel, S. M. (2008). Open hearts build lives:

Positive emotions, induced through loving-kindness meditation, build consequential personal resources. *Journal of Personal and Social Psychology, 95,* 1045–1062.

PAGE 65:   **". . . the heart breaks and the words fall in":** Moyers, W., & Ketcham, K. (2006). *Broken: My story of addiction and redemption* (frontmatter, quoted from *The Politics of the Brokenhearted* by Parker J. Palmer). New York: Viking Press.

CHAPTER 11
Self-Compassionate Motivation

PAGE 77:   **. . . drive needed to make changes or reach our goals:** Gilbert, P. P., McEwan, K. K., Gibbons, L. L., Chotai, S. S., Duarte, J. J., & Matos, M. M. (2012). Fears of compassion and happiness in relation to alexithymia, mindfulness, and self-criticism. *Psychology and Psychotherapy: Theory, Research and Practice, 85*(4), 374–390.

PAGE 78:   **. . . are less likely to fear failure:** Neff, K. D., Hseih, Y., & Dejitthirat, K. (2005). Self-compassion, achievement goals, and coping with academic failure. *Self and Identity, 4,* 263–287.

         . . . more likely to try again when they do fail: Neely, M. E., Schallert, D. L., Mohammed, S. S., Roberts, R. M., & Chen, Y. (2009). Self-kindness when facing stress: The role of self-compassion, goal regulation, and support in college students well-being. *Motivation and Emotion, 33,* 88–97.

         . . . persist in their efforts to keep learning: Breines, J. G., & Chen, S. (2012). Self-compassion increases self-improvement motivation. *Personality and Social Psychology Bulletin, 38*(9), 1133–1143.

PAGE 83:   **. . . internal family systems model of Richard Schwartz:** Schwartz, R. (1994). *Internal family systems therapy.* New York: Guilford Press.

CHAPTER 12
Self-Compassion and Our Bodies

PAGE 85:   **. . . standards of female beauty are so high:** Grogan, S. (2016). *Body image: Understanding body dissatisfaction in men, women and children.* London: Taylor & Francis.

PAGE 86:   **. . . powerful antidote to body dissatisfaction:** Braun, T. D., Park, C. L., & Gorin, A. (2016). Self-compassion, body image, and disordered eating: A review of the literature. *Body Image, 17,* 117–131.

         . . . help us appreciate our bodies as they are: Albertson, E. R., Neff, K. D., & Dill-Shackleford, K. E. (2014). Self-compassion and body dissatisfaction in women: A randomized controlled trial of a brief meditation intervention. *Mindfulness, 6*(3), 444–454.

CHAPTER 13
Stages of Progress

PAGE 96:   "We can still be crazy . . .": Chödrön, P. (1991/2001). *The wisdom of no escape and the path of loving-kindness*. Boston: Shambhala, p. 4.

"The goal of practice is to become a compassionate mess": Nairn, R. (2009, September). Lecture (part of Foundation Training in Compassion), Kagyu Samye Ling Monastery, Dumfriesshire, Scotland.

CHAPTER 14
Living Deeply

PAGE 100:   . . . deeply held ideals that guide us and give meaning to our lives: Hayes, S. C., Strosahl, K. D., & Wilson, K. G. (2011). *Acceptance and commitment therapy: The process and practice of mindful change* (2nd ed.). New York: Guilford Press.

PAGE 101:   . . . such as freedom, spiritual growth, exploration, or artistic expression: For a list of more than 50 common core values, see *http://jamesclear.com/core-values*.

PAGE 107:   Thich Nhat Hanh says, "No mud, no lotus": Nhat Hahn, T. (2014). *No mud, no lotus: The art of transforming suffering*. Berkeley, CA: Parallax Press.

CHAPTER 15
Being There for Others without Losing Ourselves

PAGE 110:   . . . *mirror neurons:* Rizzolatti, G., Fogassi, L., & Gallese, V. (2006). Mirrors in the mind. *Scientific American, 295*(5), 54–61.

. . . resonating with the emotions of others: Lloyd, D., Di Pellegrino, G., & Roberts, N. (2004). Vicarious responses to pain in anterior cingulate cortex: Is empathy a multisensory issue? *Cognitive, Affective, and Behavioral Neuroscience, 4*(2), 270–278.

CHAPTER 16
Meeting Difficult Emotions

PAGE 115:   . . . five stages of acceptance when meeting difficult emotions: Germer, C. K. (2009). *The mindful path to self-compassion: Freeing yourself from destructive thoughts and emotions*. New York: Guilford Press.

PAGE 116:   Research shows that when we label difficult emotions: Creswell, J. D., Way, B. M., Eisenberger, N. I., & Lieberman, M. D. (2007). Neural correlates of dispositional mindfulness during affect labeling. *Psychosomatic Medicine, 69*, 560–565.

CHAPTER 17

Self-Compassion and Shame

PAGE 121:   . . . food, clothing, shelter, and connection: Lieberman, M. D. (2014). *Social: Why our brains are wired to connect.* Oxford, UK: Oxford University Press.

. . . shame is feeling bad about ourselves: Tangney, J. P., & Dearing, R. L. (2003). *Shame and guilt.* New York: Guilford Press.

PAGE 122:   . . . self-compassion allows us to experience our feelings: Johnson, E. A., & O'Brien, K. A. (2013). Self-compassion soothes the savage ego-threat system: Effects on negative affect, shame, rumination, and depressive symptoms. *Journal of Social and Clinical Psychology, 32*(9), 939–963.

. . . negative core beliefs that lie at the root of shame: Dozois, D. J., & Beck, A. T. (2008). Cognitive schemas, beliefs and assumptions. *Risk Factors in Depression, 1,* 121–143.

CHAPTER 18

Self-Compassion in Relationships

PAGE 130:   "Hell is other people": Sartre, J. (1989). *No exit and three other plays* (S. Gilbert, Trans.). New York: Vintage.

Our capacity for emotional resonance: Decety, J., & Ickes, W. (2011). *The social neuroscience of empathy.* Cambridge, MA: MIT Press.

. . . *downward spiral* of negative emotions: Garland, E. L., Fredrickson, B., Kring, A. M., Johnson, D. P., Meyer, P. S., & Penn, D. L. (2010). Upward spirals of positive emotions counter downward spirals of negativity: Insights from the broaden-and-build theory and affective neuroscience on the treatment of emotion dysfunctions and deficits in psychopathology. *Clinical Psychology Review, 30*(7), 849–864.

Compassion is actually a positive emotion: Klimecki, O. M., Leiberg, S., Ricard, M., & Singer, T. (2013). Differential pattern of functional brain plasticity after compassion and empathy training. *Social Cognitive and Affective Neuroscience, 9*(6), 873–879.

PAGE 131:   . . . happier and more satisfying romantic relationships: Neff, K. D., & Beretvas, S. N. (2013). The role of self-compassion in romantic relationships. *Self and Identity, 12*(1), 78–98.

PAGE 134:   . . . adapted from the work of Paul Gilbert: Gilbert, P. (2009). Introducing compassion-focused therapy. *Advances in Psychiatric Treatment, 15,* 199–208.

CHAPTER 19
Self-Compassion for Caregivers

PAGE 138:   . . . the pain centers of our own brains become active: Lloyd, D., Di Pellegrino, G., & Roberts, N. (2004). Vicarious responses to pain in anterior cingulate cortex: Is empathy a multisensory issue? *Cognitive, Affective, and Behavioral Neuroscience, 4*(2), 270–278.

. . . experiencing distressing and intrusive thoughts: Maslach, C. (2003). Job burnout: New directions in research and intervention. *Current Directions in Psychological Science, 12*(5), 189–192.

. . . the more vulnerable they may be to caregiver fatigue: Williams, C. A. (1989). Empathy and burnout in male and female helping professionals. *Research in Nursing and Health, 12*(3), 169–178.

PAGE 139:   . . . compassion fatigue is really "empathy fatigue": Singer, T., & Klimecki, O. M. (2014). Empathy and compassion. *Current Biology, 24*(18), R875–R878.

To sense the client's private world as if it were your own: Rogers, C. (1961). *On becoming a person: A therapist's view of psychotherapy.* London: Constable, p. 248.

One research study trained people for several days: Klimecki, O. M., Leiberg, S., Ricard, M., & Singer, T. (2013). Differential pattern of functional brain plasticity after compassion and empathy training. *Social Cognitive and Affective Neuroscience, 9*(6), 873–879.

CHAPTER 20
Self-Compassion and Anger in Relationships

PAGE 144:   . . . anger has positive functions: Keltner, D., & Haidt, J. (2001). Social functions of emotions. In T. J. Mayne & G. A. Bonanno (Eds.), *Emotions: Current issues and future directions* (pp. 192–213). New York: Guilford Press.

. . . it can lead to anxiety, emotional constriction, or numbness: Dimsdale, J. E., Pierce, C., Schoenfeld, D., Brown, A., Zusman, R., & Graham, R. (1986). Suppressed anger and blood pressure: The effects of race, sex, social class, obesity, and age. *Psychosomatic Medicine, 48*(6), 430–436.

. . . which is a surefire way to become depressed: Blatt, S. J., Quinlan, D. M., Chevron, E. S., McDonald, C., & Zuroff, D. (1982). Dependency and self-criticism: Psychological dimensions of depression. *Journal of Consulting and Clinical Psychology, 50*(1), 113–124.

PAGE 145:   . . . getting angry at others for no apparent reason: Denson, T. F., Pedersen, W. C., Friese, M., Hahm, A., & Roberts, L. (2011). Understanding impulsive aggression: Angry rumination and reduced self-control capacity are mechanisms underlying the provocation–aggression relationship. *Personality and Social Psychology Bulletin, 37*(6), 850–862.

PAGE 145:   **Anger, bitterness, and resentment are "hard feelings":** Christensen, A., Doss, B., & Jacobson, N. S. (2014). *Reconcilable differences: Rebuild your relationship by rediscovering the partner you love—without losing yourself* (2nd ed.). New York: Guilford Press.

... **chronic anger causes chronic stress:** For the effects of stress on the body, see *www.apa.org/helpcenter/stress-body.aspx.*

Unmet needs are universal human needs: Rosenberg, M. B. (2003). *Nonviolent communication: A language of life.* Encinitas, CA: PuddleDancer Press.

CHAPTER 21
Self-Compassion and Forgiveness

PAGE 153:   **But forgiveness must involve grieving before letting go:** Luskin, F. (2002). *Forgive for good.* New York: HarperCollins.

PAGE 154:   **The researchers found that participants who were helped:** Breines, J. G., & Chen, S. (2012). Self-compassion increases self-improvement motivation. *Personality and Social Psychology Bulletin, 38*(9), 1133–1143.

CHAPTER 22
Embracing the Good

PAGE 160:   **it actively *generates positive emotions:*** Singer, T., & Klimecki, O. M. (2014). Empathy and compassion. *Current Biology, 24*(18), R875–R878.

The psychological term for this is *negativity bias:* Rozin, P., & Royzman, E. B. (2001). Negativity bias, negativity dominance, and contagion. *Personality and Social Psychology Review, 5*(4), 296–320.

"Velcro for bad experiences and Teflon for good ones": Hanson, R. (2009). *Buddha's brain: The practical neuroscience of happiness, love, and wisdom.* Oakland, CA: New Harbinger.

... ***intentionally* recognize and absorb positive experiences:** Hanson, R. (2013). *Hardwiring happiness: The practical science of reshaping your brain—and your life.* New York: Random House.

PAGE 161:   ... **"broaden-and-build" theory:** Fredrickson, B. L. (2004). The broaden-and-build theory of positive emotions. *Philosophical Transactions of the Royal Society B: Biological Sciences, 359*(1449), 1367–1378.

When one door of happiness closes: Keller, H. (2000). *To love this life: Quotations by Helen Keller.* New York: AFB Press.

Savoring involves mindful awareness of the *experience* of pleasure: Bryant, F.

B., & Veroff, J. (2007). *Savoring: A new model of positive experience.* Hillsdale, NJ: Erlbaum.

. . . simply taking the time to notice: Jose, P. E., Lim, B. T., & Bryant, F. B. (2012). Does savoring increase happiness?: A daily diary study. *Journal of Positive Psychology, 7*(3), 176–187.

. . . being grateful for the good things in our lives: Emmons, R. A. (2007). *Thanks!: How the new science of gratitude can make you happier.* Boston: Houghton Mifflin Harcourt.

PAGE 162: **. . . gratitude is also strongly linked to happiness:** Krejtz, I., Nezlek, J. B., Michnicka, A., Holas, P., & Rusanowska, M. (2016). Counting one's blessings can reduce the impact of daily stress. *Journal of Happiness Studies, 17*(1), 25–39.

"One key to knowing joy is to be easily pleased": Nepo, M. (2011). *The book of awakening: Having the life you want by being present to the life you have.* Newburyport, MA: Conari Press, p. 23.

James Baraz tells this wonderful story: Baraz, J., & Alexander, S. (2010). *Awakening joy: 10 steps that will put you on the road to real happiness.* New York: Bantam. Also see the video of James Baraz's mother, "Confessions of a Jewish Mother: How My Son Ruined My Life," at *www.youtube.com/watch?v=FRbL46mWx9w.*

Sense and Savor Walk: This practice is based on an exercise developed by Bryant & Veroff (2007), who found that walking in this way for one week significantly increased happiness.

PAGE 163: **"To live is so startling . . .":** Dickinson, E. (1872). Dickinson–Higginson correspondence, late 1872. Dickinson Electronic Archives. Institute for Advanced Technology in the Humanities (IATH), University of Virginia. Retrieved February 8, 2018, from *http://archive.emilydickinson.org/correspondence/higginson/l381.html.*

PAGE 164: **. . . an additional benefit of mindful eating:** Godsey, J. (2013). The role of mindfulness-based interventions in the treatment of obesity and eating disorders: An integrative review. *Complementary Therapies in Medicine, 21*(4), 430–439.

PAGE 165: **. . . research shows that "counting your blessings":** For a review of this research, see Emmons, R. A. (2007). *Thanks!: How the new science of gratitude can make you happier.* Boston: Houghton Mifflin Harcourt.

CHAPTER 23
Self-Appreciation

PAGE 167: **We can apply the three components of self-compassion:** Neff, K. (2011). *Self-compassion: The proven power of being kind to yourself.* New York: William Morrow.

. . . best-selling author and spiritual teacher Marianne Williamson: Williamson, M. (1996). *A return to love: Reflections on the principles of "A course in miracles."* San Francisco: Harper One.

Practices and Exercises

The symbol 🎧 denotes that an audio recording to complement this exercise is available at *www.guilford.com/neff-materials*.

Index

Note. *f* following a page number indicates a figure.

About the Authors

Kristin Neff, PhD, is Associate Professor of Human Development and Culture at the University of Texas at Austin and a pioneer in the field of self-compassion research. She is the author of the book *Self-Compassion* (for the general public) as well as the audio program *Self-Compassion: Step by Step* and has published numerous academic articles. She lectures and offers workshops worldwide. Together with Christopher Germer, Dr. Neff hosts an eight-hour online course, "The Power of Self-Compassion"; they are also the authors of *Teaching the Mindful Self-Compassion Program* (for professionals). Her website is *www.self-compassion.org.*

Christopher Germer, PhD, has a private practice in mindfulness- and compassion-based psychotherapy in Arlington, Massachusetts, and is a part-time Lecturer on Psychiatry at Harvard Medical School/Cambridge Health Alliance. He is a founding faculty member of the Institute for Meditation and Psychotherapy and of the Center for Mindfulness and Compassion. His books include *The Mindful Path to Self-Compassion* (for the general public) and *Wisdom and Compassion in Psychotherapy* and *Mindfulness and Psychotherapy, Second Edition* (for professionals). Dr. Germer lectures and leads workshops internationally. His website is *www. chrisgermer.com.*

List of Audio Files

Chapter	Track Number	Title	Run Time	Voice
Ch. 4	1	Self-Compassion Break	5:20	Kristin Neff
	2	Self-Compassion Break	12:21	Christopher Germer
Ch. 6	3	Affectionate Breathing	21:28	Kristin Neff
	4	Affectionate Breathing	18:24	Christopher Germer
Ch. 9	5	Loving-Kindness for a Loved One	17:08	Kristin Neff
	6	Loving-Kindness for a Loved One	14:47	Christopher Germer
Ch. 10	7	Finding Loving-Kindness Phrases	23:02	Christopher Germer
	8	Loving-Kindness for Ourselves	20:40	Christopher Germer
Ch. 12	9	Compassionate Body Scan	23:55	Kristin Neff
	10	Compassionate Body Scan	43:36	Christopher Germer
Ch. 15	11	Giving and Receiving Compassion	20:48	Kristin Neff
	12	Giving and Receiving Compassion	21:20	Christopher Germer
Ch. 16	13	Working with Difficult Emotions	16:01	Kristin Neff
	14	Working with Difficult Emotions	16:09	Christopher Germer
Ch. 18	15	Compassionate Friend	18:09	Kristin Neff
	16	Compassionate Friend	15:05	Christopher Germer
Ch. 19	17	Compassion with Equanimity	14:38	Christopher Germer

The tracks are available to download or stream from The Guilford Press website at *www.guilford.com/neff-materials.*

TERMS OF USE FOR DOWNLOADABLE AUDIO FILES